EXPANDING THE ROLE OF THE NURSE

The Scope of Professional Practice

Edited by

GEOFFREY HUNT

BSc, MLitt, PhD
Director
European Centre for Professional Ethics
Institute of Health and Rehabilitation
University of East London

PAUL WAINWRIGHT

SRN, DipN, DipANS, MSc, RNT
Senior Lecturer
The Mid and West Wales College of Nursing and Midwifery
University College of Swansea

OXFORD

BLACKWELL SCIENTIFIC PUBLICATIONS

LONDON EDINBURGH BOSTON

MELBOURNE PARIS BERLIN VIENNA

© 1994 by
Blackwell Scientific Publications
Editorial Offices:
Osney Mead, Oxford OX2 0EL
25 John Street, London WC1N 2BL
23 Ainslie Place, Edinburgh EH3 6AJ
238 Main Street, Cambridge,
  Massachusetts 02142, USA
54 University Street, Carlton,
  Victoria 3053, Australia

Other Editorial Offices:
Librairie Arnette SA
1, rue de Lille
75007 Paris
France

Blackwell Wissenschafts-Verlag GmbH
Düsseldorfer Str. 38
D-10707 Berlin
Germany

Blackwell MZV
Feldgasse 13
A-1238 Wien
Austria

First published 1994

Set by DP Photosetting, Aylesbury, Bucks
Printed and bound in Great Britain by
Hartnolls Ltd, Bodmin, Cornwall

DISTRIBUTORS

Marston Book Services Ltd
PO Box 87
Oxford OX2 0DT
(*Orders*: Tel: 0865 791155
         Fax: 0865 791927
         Telex: 837515)

USA
Blackwell Scientific Publications, Inc.
238 Main Street
Cambridge, MA 02142
(*Orders*: Tel: 800 759-6102
         617 876-7000)

Canada
Times Mirror Professional
Publishing, Ltd
130 Flaska Drive
Markham, Ontario L6G 1B8
(*Orders*: Tel: 800 268-4178)
         416 470-6739)

Australia
Blackwell Scientific Publications Pty Ltd
54 University Street,
Carlton, Victoria 3053
(*Orders*: Tel: 03 347-5552)

British Library
Cataloguing in Publication Data

A catalogue record for this book is available
from the British Library

ISBN 0–632–03604–4

Library of Congress
Cataloging in Publication Data

Expanding the role of the nurse : the scope
  of professional practice / edited by
  Geoffrey Hunt, Paul Wainwright.
    p. cm.
  Includes bibliographical references
and index.
  ISBN 0-632-03604-4
  1. Nurse practitioners—Great Britain.
2. Nurse practitioners. 3. Nursing—
Practice—Great Britain. 4. Nursing—
Practice. I. Hunt, Geoffrey, 1947–
II. Wainwright, Paul.
  [DNLM: 1. Nursing. WY 16 E94 1994]
RT82.8.E97 1994
610.73'06'9—dc20
DNLM/DLC
for Library of Congress   93-46835
                                    CIP

Contents

Contents

List of Contributors

SARAH ANDREWS MSc, PGCEA, RN, DN, CPT, DNT, Partner, Nursing First, Primary Health Care and Community Nursing Consultants, Canterbury.

PETER ASHWORTH BSc(Tech), PhD, FBPsS, CPsychol, Reader in Applied Social Studies, School of Health and Community Studies, Sheffield Hallam University.

GEORGE CASTLEDINE RGN, RNT, BA(Hons), MSc, DipSoc Stud, FRCN, Professor and Head of Nursing and Community Health, University of Central England, Birmingham.

BRIDGIT DIMOND MA, LLB, DSA, AHSM, Barrister at Law, Emeritus Professor of the University of Glamorgan.

WINNIE EVANS DipGerontology, SRN, RCNT, Lecturer/Practitioner, Queen Charlotte's College of Health and Science, Hammersmith Hospital, London.

GEOFFREY HUNT BSc, MLitt, PhD, Director, European Centre for Professional Ethics, Institute of Health and Rehabilitation, University of East London.

GARY JONES RGN, OND, DipN(Lond), FETC, is a freelance nurse consultant and lecturer based at Grays, Essex.

DIRK KEYZER RGN, DANS, MSc, PhD, Professor of Community Health Nursing, Faculty of Health and Behavioural Sciences, Deakin University, Australia.

TOM LAST RGN, ENB100(Cert), Senior Nurse, Resource Management Department, Gwynedd Acute Hospitals Unit, Bangor, North Wales.

PAUL MORRISON RMN, RGN, BA, PGCE, PhD, AFBPsS, CPsychol, Lecturer, School of Nursing Studies, University of Wales College of Medicine.

EIRA ROWLEY RGN, DipSocAdmin, DNCert, PWT, Cert Health Ed, CHNT, DNT, RNT, MA (Ed) Professional Adviser, Primary Health Care, Welsh National Board for Nursing, Midwifery and Health Visiting, Cardiff.

NIGEL SELF RGN, ENB100(Cert), Staff Nurse, Intensive Care Unit, St Mary's Hospital Trust, Isle of Wight.

LOUISE SILVERTON BSc, SRN SCM, MSc, MTD, Head of Maternal and Child Health, Nightingale and Guy's College of Health, London.

PAUL WAINWRIGHT SRN, DipN, DipANS, MSc, RNT, Senior Lecturer, The Mid and West Wales College of Nursing and Midwifery, University College of Swansea.

Preface

This book has its origins in a discussion between Paul Wainwright, Tom Last, Nigel Self and Geoffrey Hunt held at the National Centre for Nursing and Midwifery Ethics, at the Hammersmith Hospital in 1991. Last and Self were at the time undertaking a national survey on the extended role of the nurse in intensive care units (Chapter 8). A literature search showed up very little besides the official documents on the important issue of the changing role of the nurse. A decision was made to work on a book which would draw the wider attention of the profession to the survey while examining other dimensions and clinical areas of role extension. We were intrigued by the suggestiveness of a distinction between role *extension* and role *expansion* and wanted to get clearer about its meaning and ramifications.

Paul Wainwright qualified as a nurse, was until recently a professional adviser with the Welsh National Board and is now working in higher education, while Geoffrey Hunt is a social philosopher. We hoped that this novel combination of editorial wisdom would result in a book which would be not only informative and topical but questioning and critical. Some of the questions posed are quite fundamental, perhaps more fundamental than is customary in nursing studies. If nursing is to be liberated from its nineteenth century shackles and come alive to the dramatic changes now occurring in health care delivery, then fundamental questions need to be asked about the very nature of nursing, its role in society and its future.

In 1993 the National Centre for Nursing and Midwifery Ethics moved to the University of East London, and changed its name to the European Centre for Professional Ethics. This resulted in some delay in bringing out the book. However, without the support of the University, particularly Professor John Neville, Dean of the Institute of Health and Rehabilitation, and Mrs Linda Hanford, Head of the Department of Health Studies, the book might never have seen the light of day. We are grateful to them.

Thanks are also due to those bodies which have given us permission to reproduce official documents and previously published work. The section headed 'The Code' in Geoffrey Hunt's contribution in Chapter 2 appeared in the *Nursing Times* on 17 June 1992. This is reproduced by kind permission of the *Nursing Times*. In the Appendices, *The Scope of Professional Practice* and part of the 'PREPP Report', are reproduced with the permission of the United Kingdom Central Council for Nursing, Midwifery and Health Visiting; and 'The Extending Role of the Nurse' and a section of the 'Report of the Advisory Group on Nurse Prescribing' are Crown copyright. They are reproduced with the permission of the Controller of Her Majesty's Stationery Office.

Introduction

A wind of change is blowing across nursing in the United Kingdom, Europe and beyond. Where this wind blows and whether nursing should sail with it or tack against it are still not clear. What is growing clear is that nursing will become more diversified in character, less monolithic and more specialised than before.

Under the impact of new economic and social policies, administrative and managerial reorganisation, and technological developments, nursing is struggling to define its own character, its own kind of knowledge and its own professional goals and standards.

Professional nursing will have to define itself within a wider social trend. All the occupations are on a kind of escalator. Tasks which were the responsibility of a small echelon of highly placed individuals are increasingly carried out further down the pyramid. Alternatively, one could think of the proliferating techniques undertaken in a modern industrial and bureaucratic society moving down the escalator into ever widening circles of the population.

Ever since its origins nursing has been engaged in a process in which some tasks have come to be regarded as menial and not part of nursing, so that less qualified or unqualified staff have taken them on. For example, most nurses no longer regard cleaning as a nursing duty, but it was their duty in the past. Even Florence Nightingale saw cleaning as part of the nurses' duty to maintain hygiene and protect patients from harm (Gray 1992). Lower paid and unqualified staff now clean. Concurrently, doctors came to see some of their tasks as non-medical and a proper part of nursing, while they accepted as part of the medical routine tasks previously left to medical specialists such as surgeons (Knott 1985).

This process continues in the current phenomenon of 'role expansion' in nursing, although it is perhaps qualitatively different from the past in important respects due to the far-reaching economic, administrative and ideological changes currently being exacted by governments.

The expanding role of the nurse is an issue because of a unique historic conjuncture of professional developments, radical reforms in health care delivery as a whole, technological advances and the growth of nursing research and knowledge, and cultural, educational and legal changes.

Nursing has undergone a natural process of growth in its scope of responsibilities through medical delegation, through having to cope with emergency situations and through advances in nursing technique. Pressure for change has grown by accretion. A striking case is that of legislation to enable nurse prescribing. It is not entirely new, but rather the result of the pressure of actual practice which has built up historically until the existing legal and administrative framework is patently outdated and unduly restrictive. Following a survey of nurses a Department of Health Report says, 'Most nurses regarded prescribing as the legitimisation of the status quo rather than an advance in their professional standing' (DoH 1991a).

The regulatory body for nurses, midwives and health visitors, The United Kingdom Central Council for Nursing, Midwifery and Health Visiting (UKCC), has also had to respond to such changes, for if it had not it would have lost the respect of the profession and ultimately could have lost control of it. The UKCC's document *The Scope of Professional Practice* (UKCC 1992 and see Appendix I in this volume) is quite innovative, and indeed formulates in official terms the rationale for a book of this kind. But as the *Nursing Times* points out, 'As is often the case with official guidance, the printed document lags behind the cutting edge of clinical practice' (Carlisle 1992).

The development of nursing and the changing context in which nursing takes place had reached a point at which nursing itself had to recognise the need to enlarge its scope.

'The days are over when a nurse trained to carry out defibrillation in an intensive care unit can be prevented from defibrillating a patient in a neighbouring care of the elderly unit. The night sister traipsing from ward to ward because she alone is trained to give intravenous drugs will be a thing of the past. Patients should no longer have to be kept waiting for antibiotics because the doctor is still in theatre. Men needing catheterisation need not be brought into hospital merely because the district nurse lacks the authority to do the job herself' (Carlisle 1992).

Some Government initiatives in the area of nursing and related professions may appear to lead, but really represent a recognition of a process of maturation in the professions themselves. Thus the latest Department of Health document on nursing, *A Vision for the Future*, speaks of a need for 'a flexible, knowledgeable, and skilful response from nurses, midwives and health visitors to the needs of users and their carers.' (DoH 1993). It states that practitioners must consider how to develop their practice; providers should be able to identify education that promotes such development and also demonstrate three areas in which clinical practice has improved as a result of research findings. At the same time employers should be able to show how potential leaders and managers are identified and developed.

It is one thing to recognise the potential that nursing has itself developed, while making exhortations to realise that potential, and quite another to facilitate implementation. Difficult questions have to be answered as to the consistency of economic and social policies. Are the economic, managerial, administrative structures being redesigned to facilitate the kind of nursing role expansion which would benefit patients?

New forces are now at work, such as the increase in private sector nursing. What will be the character of this in relation to public sector styles and structures? Will nursing become fragmented, with little unity? There are concerns that nursing role expansion really complements the Government's effort to reduce the number of hours worked by junior doctors, turning nurses into low-cost 'surrogate doctors' (Giles 1993; DoH 1991b).

The issue is not clear. Thus, one junior doctor has asserted that 'Many of the tasks performed by junior doctors have nothing to do with their training ... tasks [which] have no long-term educational value to the doctor; junior doctors perform them on a learning curve which means that patients receive less than optimal care'. He gives the example of senior house officers training to enter general practice who are put to work in the labour suite where they are required to suture episiotomies, interpret cardiotocographs, and perform artificial membrane ruptures (Ashcroft 1992; also see Pogmore 1992).

Of course, it does not follow that because certain doctors should not do certain tasks, nurses or midwives should do them. The pertinent consideration here surely is that role expansion should be led by patients' needs rather than by medical delegation or costsaving.

Everyone is aware of the managerial preoccupation with cost and suspicions are aroused. For example, nurse practitioners may be seen as a cheap option to general practitioners. But while some GPs see nurse practitioners as a threat, others see them as a means of enhancing their own medical practice, allowing them to expand their role in novel directions.

This echoes a debate going on a few steps down the escalator – the debate about health care assistants. Are they a threat or a boon to nursing? There is evidence that in the current economic climate registered nurses are having to take jobs as care assistants (*Nursing Times* 1993). On the other hand, the development of a large body of care assistants, with vocational qualifications, has been seen by some as an opportunity for the advancement of nursing care by freeing up nursing time. A lot depends on what advantages the nursing profession itself takes of the situation as it expands its scope of practice.

The influence on nursing of advances in scientific understanding and technology in the last decade, whether directly or indirectly through medical practice, should not be underestimated. For example, it is now common to find on almost any ward the use of intravenous administration of drugs, together with the use of indwelling cannulae and central or Hickman lines. This advance breeds a general familiarity which soon poses the question of whether nurses should be involved.

Naturally, this has resulted in nurses seizing and developing a scientific territory of their own. As Allman puts it: 'The more the distinct nature of the process of nursing is identified, the more nursing can be the subject of distinct intellectual activity, with its own academic base and research component' (Allman 1993).

Intensive care nursing is an area in which one might expect expansion to be technology-led. Last and Self conducted a survey of what tasks ICU nurses are actually undertaking and what their views on their role, and changing it, are (Chapter 8). The result is curious in so far as most nurses are keen to take on new techniques but are diffident about doing so without certification. This runs counter to recent official thinking.

Here it appears that the UKCC's 'Scope' document is both following changes in nurse practice and leading changes in nurse thinking. It breaks with the idea of certificating every task which 'extends' the role and it opens the way to a self-propelling growth of nursing responsibilities. Certainly the UKCC is playing its part, together with professional organisations, universities and nurses themselves in bringing about a *cultural* change in nursing to match wider changes in society at large.

It is undeniable that the attitudes, expectations and beliefs of society in relation to health, illness, childbirth, old age, disability and so on are changing quite dramatically. The biomedical model is losing some of its legitimacy. The role of the nurse has to adapt to such transformations.

Formal education is an obvious arena in which critical thinking about nursing is finding a new lease of life. While changes in the goals and delivery of education (Project 2000, PREPP, programmes in higher education) have been driven by developments in the practice, organisation and context of nursing, there can be little doubt that the higher education environment will increasingly drive developments in the profession.

Of course, role expansion need not be academically led – it should be experience-led if it is to be responsive to patients' changing patterns of needs and values. Invaluable nursing experience spread far and wide through our health care institutions, whether in hospitals or the community, is not always tapped. Thus, the issue of enrolled nurses taking part in the tidal wave of skills enhancement has still perhaps not been adequately addressed with regard to the undervaluing of their experience and their access to appropriate courses.

More attention is perhaps being given to advanced and specialist practice which, as Castledine points out in this volume, has at last been recognised in the UK. The Royal College of Nursing, for example, has risen to the challenge with a new nurse practitioners' diploma course. The principal tutor on the course is reported as saying, 'We set out to create autonomous practitioners who would be able to see patients with undiagnosed conditions and assess and treat them accordingly' (Simon 1992).

Education for practice nurses is also beginning to take shape, although it is still true that 'A barrier to the development of a well-defined role for practice nurses has been the lack of a distinct training structure' (Traynor 1991). For example, if screening of the elderly and health promotion are to be regarded as standard skills of nurses working in GP practices, then they ought to have a formal training in these skills (RCN 1984, 1991).

Still, which way is the wind blowing? Many of the educational changes we are seeing are shaped by an economic ideology, and go hand in hand with the industrial/market model of public welfare provision currently holding sway. Ashworth and Morrison say in Chapter 3 that there is a tendency to prioritise technical skill over nursing care for the person. This manifests itself in the way the competence model underwrites nurse education, with its emphasis on discrete, measurable elements of behaviour.

The expanding role of nurses has also given rise to concerns about their legal status. In Chapter 4 Dimond asks a number of germane questions, such as: What legal restrictions are there on who performs what? How are competency and liability determined? How do these issues relate to falling standards and inadequate resources and the demands of employers?

Extension or expansion?

There were two ways the increasing responsibilities of nurses could have been recognised. One way was growth by mechanical addition of parts (extension) and the other way was organic growth of the whole (expansion). The UKCC has chosen the latter, as is fitting for the development of a profession.

In the 'Scope' document the UKCC rejects the notion of 'role extension' – the notion that any task which goes beyond what is learned in pre-registration training requires official sanction by certification. Highly skilled nurses, under this system, could end up with quite a collection of certificates. On the one hand, any particular certificate might not be recognised when they moved from one workplace to another while, on the other hand, if they did not have a particular certificate they might be prevented from carrying out a procedure, even though they were highly skilled in it. The UKCC states:

'The Council considers that the terms 'extended' or 'extending' roles which have been associated with this system are no longer suitable since they limit, rather than extend, the parameters of practice. As a result, many practitioners have been prevented from fulfilling their potential for the benefit of patients. The Council also believes that a concentration on 'activities' can detract from the importance of holistic nursing care.' (UKCC 1992)

The 'Scope' document thus manifests a shift from attempting to direct the specific to giving guidance on the general, from external control to professional discretion. Nurses no longer have to ask themselves whether they have proved through some formal procedure that they can do a particular task. On the other hand, it is not a matter of simply doing anything they feel confident to do. They have to pose to themselves some general questions.

These general questions are set out by the UKCC as 'Principles for adjusting the Scope of Practice'. To paraphrase: nurses must always remember that the point of their work lies in the needs and interests of the patient, and in serving those needs and interests must recognise their limitations while trying to push back those limitations in a way that is safe, ethical and does not compromise or fragment practice, and accept their personal accountability for their actions, avoiding inappropriate delegation.

Does role expansion represent a real quantum leap in practice? If so, how exactly? The key to this is *autonomy*. If role expansion is about anything it is about nurses taking their *own* initiative, doing their own thinking and making their own decisions based on their own experience and education, to improve practice for the benefit of patients and clients.

An illustration of how a specific extension of nursing practice provides opportunities for expanding nursing, rather than just tagging on another technical task, is given by Andrews in Chapter 5. Nurse prescribing, she says, provides 'the greatest opportunity to combine this intervention with health education. The prescribed product is introduced on the understanding that the end goal is self-care or carer action...'. Keyser too, in Chapter 6 says, 'Role extension is inevitably linked to advances in medical technology, whereas role expansion appears to be more likely to succeed in community based health-orientated services'.

Role expansion then is not merely about extending the list of techniques that nurses, midwives and health visitors have at their disposal, but neither is it necessarily against such extension. It is about enhancing care of the needy person in social context, and accepting new responsibilities if they represent a means to *that* end.

References

Allman S. (1993) 1993 and beyond. In *Nursing: The European Dimension* (eds S. Quinn & S. Russell), p 38. Scutari, London.

Ashcroft J. (1992) Rising to the challenge. *Nursing Times* **88**(37), 30.

Carlisle D. (1992) Scope for extensions. *Nursing Times* **88**(37), pp. 26–8.

DoH (1991a) *Nurse Prescribing, Final Report: A Cost Benefit Study*. Department of Health, London.

DoH (1991b) *Doctors in Training: A New Deal*. Department of Health, London.

DoH (1993) *A Vision for the Future*. Department of Health, London.

Giles S. (1993) Passing the buck. *Nursing Times* **89**(28), 42–43.

Gray J. (1992) Sweeping changes. *Nursing Standard* **6**(19), 22–23.

Knott L. (1985) Case for nurse practitioner. *Pulse*, 12 October, 33.

Nursing Times (1993) Nurses forced to take care assistant jobs, News report. *Nursing Times* **89**(28), 8.

Pogmore J. R. (1992) Role of the senior house officer in the labour ward. *British Journal of Obstetrics and Gynaecology* **99**(3) 180–181.

RCN (1984) *Training Needs of Practice Nurses: Report of Steering Group*. Royal College of Nursing, London.

RCN (1991) *Standards of Care for Practice Nursing*. Royal College of Nursing, London.

Simon P. (1992) Pioneer spirit. *Nursing Times* **88**(30), 16.

Traynor M. (1991) Practice nurses: at the crossroads. *Nursing Standard* **5**(51), 33–35.

United Kingdom Central Council for Nursing, Midwifery and Health Visiting (1992) *The Scope of Professional Practice*. UKCC, London.

Part I
General Themes

Chapter 1
Professionalism and the Concept of Role Extension

Introduction

It seems as if there has not been a time, at least in this century, when the nature of nursing and the role of the nurse have not been the subject of discussion and contention. By tradition nursing has been seen as a dependent occupation, the nurse being expected to be the ears and eyes of the doctor, loyally carrying out instructions and faithfully reporting back. A nurse was expected to be 'punctual, good tempered, obedient, and loyal to all rules as the foundation of her work'. She should also remember 'what is due to authority' and 'must ever remember that discipline and obedience are the keynote to satisfactory and efficient work in life'. Among other things the nurse should 'dust the sick room, wash and cleanse all utensils used by the patient, and never ... refuse to do domestic work in exceptional cases of extreme illness, infectious disease or straitened circumstances' (Ashdown 1943).

Changing social norms and mores have meant that the degree of servility implied by descriptions such as Ashdown's has been steadily eroded over the years. However, there has been a more fundamental shift in attitudes and approaches to the division of labour in more recent years, particularly since the 1960s, with a burst of activity in the 1980s. Indeed, such has been the pace and significance of the change in thinking on the part of at least some nurse leaders that writers such as Salvage (1992) have coined the phrase 'The New Nursing' to describe what they see as a movement. Characteristics of the New Nursing include attempts to redefine the nurse's role in order to assert its unique contribution to healing, the challenging of assumptions about nursing's subordination to medicine, and the idea of replacing a bureaucratic occupation with a profession.

This chapter will consider some aspects of the development of nursing as a profession with claims to an increasingly independent function, and within this context will examine notions of role extension, expansion, and the scope of professional practice.

3

The nature of nursing work

Nursing as we know it today has its origins in the early nineteenth century, although we can trace it further back to the middle ages (Buckenham & McGrath 1983). Nursing as an occupation developed as an extension of the work women were expected to do in the home (McKee & Lessof 1992; Reverby 1987), with nurses viewed as relatively unskilled doctors' helpers. Right up to the present nursing has been seen as subordinate to and dominated by medicine, to the extent that for many years doctors had a key role in deciding the content of the nursing curriculum and in the appointment of nursing staff; it is still quite common to hear consultant medical staff talking of 'my nurses'.

As Buckenham and McGrath (1983) remind us, Nightingale lifted nursing from its Dickensian image of a sordid duty, performed by the lowest class in the community, and reintroduced the idea of nursing as a vocation, a service of special value in the eyes of God. Along with this came stereotypical Victorian upper class values, with a training that stressed the development of character rather than skills, and obedience rather than reasoning. The domestic origins of the role persisted through a relationship which placed the nurse as an extension of the doctor's 'good wife', combining the virtues of obedience and subservience with the role of kind and compassionate mother in relation to the patients, and the firm but kindly discipline of the lady of the house in relation to domestic staff. Much of this view of nursing persisted well into the twentieth century.

As medicine became more technical and more scientific, nurses increasingly took on skills and procedures that had once been the preserve of doctors, and doctors came to appreciate the value of 'patient, obedient helpers who could in no way be seen to be competing in the medical field' (Buckenham & McGrath 1983). However, the dependence of nursing on medicine to take the main responsibility for decision making continued. Nurses had become adept at suggesting a course of action to a doctor in a way which allowed him to think that he had initiated it (the 'doctor–nurse game' described by Stein in 1967). However, the very fact that nurses used such strategies suggests that there was no great desire to challenge medical authority or to seek autonomy. Indeed, as Davies (1976) suggests, nursing saw considerable benefits in this dependent relationship.

Not only have nurses been seen as dependent upon doctors and therefore shielded from responsibility, but there has also been a long tradition of hierarchical structures within nursing. Historically this can be seen in nursing's roots in domestic service, the church and the military. More recently it has been perpetuated through organisational systems of matrons, assistant matrons and ward sisters, and from the late 1960s with the introduction of the Salmon management structure (Ministry of Health 1966).

Nursing is seen as a particularly stressful occupation, as Menzies (1960) describes in graphic terms:

> 'The situations likely to evoke stress in nurses are familiar. Nurses are in constant contact with people who are physically ill or injured, often seriously. The recovery of patients is not certain and will not always be complete. Nursing patients who have incurable diseases is one of the nurse's most distressing tasks. Nurses are confronted with the threat and the reality of suffering and death as few lay people are. Their work involves carrying out tasks which, by ordinary standards, are distasteful, disgusting, and frightening.'

One may not accept the full Freudian analysis of nursing work and its attendant anxiety that Menzies presents, but one cannot argue with her description of what she sees as 'the attempt to eliminate decisions by ritual task performance', involving precise instructions about the way tasks must be performed, their order and the time they must be done, 'although such precise instructions are not objectively necessary, or even wholly desirable'.

Not only are tasks reduced to rituals and procedures, but the 'psychological burden of anxiety' which might arise from making a decision, is dissipated through such strategies as elaborate checking and re-checking and the postponing of action as long as possible. Menzies observed that such checking took place even in situations where the implications 'are only of the slightest consequence ... Nurses consult not only their immediate seniors but also their juniors and nurses or other staff with whom they have no functional relationship but who just happen to be available'. Still more protection from the impact of responsibility used to be gained under traditional management arrangements from a lack of clarity about role content and boundaries within the nursing hierarchy. The structure and role system failed to define who actually was responsible for what and to whom.

A further characteristic of nursing organisation, identified by Menzies but still apparent today, is what she called 'the reduction of the impact of responsibility by delegation to superiors'. Contrary to the normal practice of delegation from superior to subordinate, in the hospital tasks are frequently forced upwards in the hierarchy, 'so that all responsibility for their performance can be disclaimed'. This practice within the nursing structure reflects the similar practice of avoiding responsibility through deference to doctors.

Is nursing a profession?

One feels almost apologetic for raising this question yet again, when so much has already been written and said on the subject. However, the problem shows no signs of going away, and in the course of a brief review of the arguments it is intended to make some points that are considered relevant to the discussion of the scope of practice.

Bayles (1989) observes that there is no generally accepted definition of the term 'profession'. Many writers have attempted to draw up lists of attributes, the presence of which is necessary for any occupational group to claim the status of profession. The most common attributes are: extensive training; a significant intellectual component or unique body of knowledge; the provision of an important service to society; some system of credentials or licensing to control admission; the organisation of members; and autonomy in their work. Different authors place more or less stress on different attributes. Etzioni for example feels that a minimum of 5 years training is required and that those groups who require less training should be classified as semi-professions (Etzioni 1969).

Friedson (1970) on the other hand suggests that a profession is an occupation that has assumed a dominant position in a division of labour, so that it gains control over the determination of the substance of its own work, and is thus autonomous and self-directing. However, he recognises the difficulty of providing one definition:

'Beyond being full-time pursuits of some significance or social prominence, it is difficult to find very much agreement on a definition of the word "profession". Virtually all self-conscious occupational groups apply it to themselves at one time or another either to flatter themselves or to try to persuade others of their importance. Occupations to which the word has been applied are thus so varied as to have nothing in common save a hunger for prestige.'

Vollmer and Mills (1966) attempt to get away from the problem of defining professions in terms of a set of necessary and sufficient attributes through the notion of the ideal type. Professionalisation can be seen as a process of evolutionary change, as an occupation changes with respect to a range of characteristics. Each characteristic is represented as a continuum along which an occupation can be placed. The extent of professionalisation can then be assessed in terms of the position of the occupation on any or all of these continua.

There is considerable debate within nursing about the status of the occupation as a profession. Sleicher (1981) takes a typical view, arguing that nursing is still less than a profession in several respects, and cites in particular the attributes of commitment, a body of knowledge, the level of education, the extent of autonomy, and the notion of service as areas in which nursing falls short. On the other hand, Cleland (1975) suggests that in the USA nursing is defined in law as a profession, pointing out that the National Labor Relations Act Section 2(12) defines 'professional employee' as:

'(a) any employee engaged in work (i) predominantly intellectual and varied in character as opposed to routine mental, manual, mechanical, or physical work; (ii) involving the consistent exercise of discretion and judgement in its performance; (iii) of such a character that the output produced or the result accomplished cannot be standardised in relation to a given period of time; (iv) requiring knowledge of an advanced type in a field of science or learning customarily acquired by a prolonged course of specialised intellectual instruction and study in an institution of higher learning or a hospital, as distinguished from a general academic education or from an apprenticeship or from training in the performance of routine mental, manual, or physical processes; or

(b) any employee, who (i) has completed the courses of specialised intellectual instruction and study described in clause (iv) of paragraph (a), and (ii) is performing related work under the supervision of a professional person to qualify himself to become a professional employee as defined in paragraph (a).'

Previous rulings have established that the registered nurse is a professional employee according to the NLRA definition.

It could be argued that it is hardly surprising that there is such comprehensive failure to arrive at a certain and consistent definition of a concept such as 'profession'. Although there is a natural human desire to discover some unity of meaning for the words and concepts we use the philosopher Wittgenstein has shown us that this search for the essence of words is mistaken (Wittgenstein 1958).

There is a natural assumption that there is something that is common to all members of a class or category, such as all tables, or all games, or all professions or all nurses. But Wittgenstein (1958) shows us that terms such as these show not unity and essence but multiplicity and difference. One has only to examine the individuals to which a general term is applied to see that there may be nothing that they all have in common and that they do not in fact share a common essence. This is not to say that such groups are arbitrary collections of things which happen to be called by the same name. Although they have no common essence they have what Wittgenstein calls 'family resemblances'.

If we examine such groups with their family resemblances we see 'a complicated network of similarities overlapping and criss-crossing: sometimes overall similarities, sometimes similarities of detail' (Wittgenstein 1958). Wittgenstein likens the development of a concept to the spinning of a thread: '... in spinning a thread we twist fibre on fibre. And the strength of the thread does not reside in the fact that some one fibre runs through its whole length, but in the overlapping of many fibres'.

Contemporary writers on nursing work who discard the notion of an attribute-based definition of a profession include Dingwall *et al.* (1988), who argue that lists of attributes tend to be vague and inconsistent, and to be compiled in order to yield particular results. Such lists also end up with very little to say about the organisation of work or of society, and seem more concerned with the ranking of occupations on some sort of prestige scale. These authors also reject the 'evolutionary process' approach, and point out that a major difficulty with the term 'profession' is that it is used in two different ways: as a folk concept which can be used by anyone to describe any occupation or activity with respect; and in the more technical sense of a label for a group of occupations.

Dingwall *et al.* (1988) suggest a more profitable line of enquiry is to ask not 'What is a profession?', but 'What kinds of occupation are there and how do they divide the work that has to be done in a society?'. The division of the workforce into occupations creates a scheme for the social classification of work. There being no necessary relationship between the categories of such a scheme, the occupations and the tasks that need doing, we can ask why it is that tasks are shared out in one way or another at different times and in different places.

Dingwall *et al.* (1988) propose a novel analogy. They suggest a comparison between the social organisation of work and the development of a city. The work that has to be done can be seen as the land on which the city is built, while the different occupations represent the buildings to be put on that land. However, cities are not static. Their boundaries are constantly changing, redevelopment is occurring all the time, and some buildings are being improved and enlarged while others are demolished and their sites used for new developments. In the same way the definition of work is continually changing. New occupations are created while others disappear or divide or fuse with others.

Dingwall *et al.* (1988) suggest that one way of seeing the Nurses Registration Act of 1919 is as a licence for a group of people to redevelop part of the city. The shape and size of the buildings that were erected under this licence were partly determined by the nature of the site and the previous development work. Developments on the site continued and the resulting changes were formalised by the new Nurses, Midwives and Health Visitors Acts of 1979 and 1992.

The role of the nurse and the scope of practice

Among the family resemblances which characterise those occupations that are generally recognised as professions is the claim on the part of members that they have control over the determination of the substance of their own work. The professional is autonomous and self-directing, and this position is maintained because society is persuaded of the trustworthiness of members, their ethical probity and knowledgeable skill, and the status of the profession as the most reliable authority on the nature of the reality with which it deals (Friedson 1970).

McKee and Lessof (1992) point out that once doctors, for example, qualify there is an implicit assumption that they are skilled in all of the tasks necessary for the diagnosis and treatment of patients under their care or that, if they are not, they will call for assistance as required. With nurses, on the other hand, it is assumed that the skill is absent unless it has been taught and tested. Kloss (1988) tells us that 'Nurses as a profession place considerable emphasis on formal training and hold that a nurse is not competent to perform a task which she has not been specifically trained to do, unlike most other professions, which recognise training acquired through practical experience'.

This attitude was reinforced by the (then) Department of Health and Social Security in its Health Circular which states that work 'which has hitherto been carried out by doctors ought therefore to be delegated to nurses only when ... the nurse has been specifically and adequately trained for the performance of the new task and she agrees to undertake it' (DHSS 1977). This position was reinforced by a later circular (DHSS, 1989) which defines the activities of nurses in terms of three categories:

(i) Those activities for which nurses are prepared in the course of their pre-registration training;

(ii) Those more specialised activities for which nurses are prepared by post-registration training. These include the activities undertaken in the community, by for example Health Visitors, District Nurses and Community Psychiatric Nurses;

(iii) Activities normally undertaken by doctors but which may be delegated in appropriate circumstances, and which may be performed by nurses with appropriate training and competence (see Appendix V).

Later in the document it is emphasised that 'the nurse's primary obligation is to the performance of nursing activities that fall within her customary professional role, i.e. within the first two categories'.

The position taken by the DHSS is fundamentally flawed in two respects. First, it assumes that there are such things as activities 'normally undertaken by doctors but which may be delegated' which by implication cannot normally be undertaken by anyone else. There are very few activities which are normally undertaken exclusively by doctors. Almost everything a doctor does, is done or can be done by somebody else, somewhere and at some time, and the same is true for nearly everything done by nurses and other health care workers. It is certainly far from clear what tasks come under the authority of a doctor such that they can effectively be delegated to another. The activities which only a doctor may perform are those controlled by statute, and these may either be delegated under specific conditions identified within the statute, or would need changes in legislation to allow their delegation. The category of 'activities normally undertaken by doctors but which may be delegated' is thus to all intents and purposes an empty category.

Second, it assumes that activities that fall within the customary role of the nurse are restricted to those that are taught in pre-registration or post-basic courses. This clearly is nonsense. Even if we grant nurses' predilection for routine tasks, written procedures, and the avoidance of responsibility and decision making, it cannot be true that having undertaken a 3-year statutory training and qualified as nurses, they are frozen in limbo and cannot take on any new activities until they have the chance to attend a formal post-basic course.

Salvage (1992) has highlighted the developments that have taken place over the last decade or so. The New Nursing is based on a new set of values and beliefs about the nature of nursing and of practice, and is directly opposed to notions of nursing as a dependent occupation. Many of the strategies described by Menzies (1960) and Davies (1976) as means by which nurses avoid responsibility or anxiety are in direct opposition to the new values. Menzies for example discusses the 'splitting up of the nurse–patient relationship', arguing that the closer and more concentrated the relationship the more likely it is that the nurse will experience anxiety as a result. The use of a task-based model of care delivery ensures that in effect the nurse 'does not nurse patients', but instead performs a small number of tasks for as many of the patients as require that particular element of care. This ensures that the nurse does not come into contact with the totality of any one patient and thus reduces the likelihood of anxiety.

Menzies (1960) goes on to describe strategies such as depersonalisation and categorisation of patients according to bed numbers and disease entities, and the denial of the significance of the individual through the wearing of uniforms and insignia. Hats, for example, are seen as a way of displaying insignia of rank or seniority and thus creating 'an operational identity between all nurses in the same category' which can help to eliminate painful and difficult decisions. She also discusses the detachment and denial of feelings, the performance of rituals, the over-use of checking and counter checking mechanisms, and the 'collusive social redistribution of responsibility', including upward delegation. Finally she discusses the avoidance of change, citing examples of 'clinging to the inappropriate familiar'.

Davies (1976) describes many of the characteristics discussed by Menzies, including the routinisation of work with an emphasis on tasks, rule following and a hierarchical structure for supervision. She recog-nises the value of such strategies for the reduction of stress and uncertainty, but offers a sociological rather than a psychological ana-lysis. She reminds us that three features of nursing, the acceptance of doctors as superior, the valuing of routines and the acceptance of a broad range of tasks, made sense in the 1860s, in the context of the Nightingale reforms, and still had advantages in 1976.

In particular, Davies (1976) emphasises the importance of the location of power and authority in the role of the matron. There could exist, under matron's close control, an 'obedient and highly useful additional labour force for a variety of tasks in the hospital', with nursing staff firmly subordinate to the authority of matron and discipline the norm. Matron became a powerful figure, while the nurse on the ward was 'a quiet and obedient follower of routine'. Davies suggests that, in addition to creating a certain set of circumstances within the workplace, strate-gies such as these may have helped nursing to gain recognition by winning public sympathy: 'Had nurses attempted to carve out for themselves a clear area of expertise rather then carrying out in an unprotesting fashion all the jobs, however humble and routine, neces-sary for patient comfort and recovery, there may have been less public sympathy and less State support'.

Davies (1976) offers three reasons for the continued adoption of such strategies. First, as we have already seen, the routinisation of work lessens stress. Second, 'routinisation of work ... can function to protect the nurse from the arbitrary whim of a superior or a doctor'. Nurses, like clerical workers, show a preference 'for rule following rather than engaging in a reciprocal negotiating process'. And thirdly, routinisation is a helpful solution when there is high turnover of staff. Newcomers are more easily familiarised with the situation when there are standardised procedures and a task-based approach. In the past nursing has had dif-ficulties recruiting staff and keeping them, so routines mean that replacements can work smoothly. All three of these arguments are open to a rather different analysis today.

To take the third, the problems of turnover, this simply is no longer a problem, for the time being at least. All the evidence suggests that the combination of the introduction of clinical grading and the recession has resulted in a far more static workforce. Indeed there is some irony in the fact that some contemporary approaches to the management of the workforce seek to recreate some aspects of high turnover because they are seen to be useful. There is an increasing interest in notions of a reduced core staff supported by occasional workers from nurse banks or agencies, or the employment of staff on part time contracts with the offer of extra hours when the workload demands; where natural turnover has reduced or disappeared there are an increasing number of nursing staff being made redundant.

The second feature, the protective nature of rule following, illustrates very clearly the lack of power and authority experienced by nursing as an occupation. Most professions do not need the existence of rules and policies to protect members from 'the arbitrary whim of a superior' (Davies 1976). This is because in the content and practice of their work they recognise no superiors and this is reinforced by professional regulation and sometimes by statute. Professionals can refer to what Rowbottom (1978) has called 'binding standards', supported by their professional association and with the threat of removal from a professional register as a sanction. Rowbottom suggests the existence of binding standards limits the extent to which an individual can be directed by superiors and the existence of such standards indicates 'a level of professional development that makes effective management by non-members of the profession difficult if not impossible'.

In the last few years we have seen a concerted attempt in some quarters to suppress the development of nursing as a profession with control over the content of its own work. As Keyzer (1992) points out, 'the nursing profession will have to acknowledge that as a major organisational power general managers have the authority to define nursing; to create new divisions of labour within the health care team; and to rethink nursing's place within the new order'.

The first of Davies' points is that routinisation of work serves to reduce stress. As Pembrey (1980) points out, the performance of work involves the worker in a series of choices or decisions about the way in which the task is to be performed or the goal achieved. This results in a mental process, the exercise of discretion, and different jobs at different levels in organisations are characterised by the amount of discretion available to the worker. Individuals are said to have a capacity for work, and that capacity in part is determined by the ability of the individual to handle the anxiety that results from the exercise of discretion.

It is clear that the institution of detailed routines and policies and the assignment of work as tasks to be performed can reduce the potential for anxiety by reducing or eliminating the element of discretion open to the individual worker. However, it would seem that an alternative approach would be to increase the ability of the worker to handle discretion by increasing his ability to deal with the choices with which he may be confronted. This could most obviously be done by increasing the level of knowledge and skill possessed by the worker and combining this knowledge and skill with appropriate experience. Such an approach would be supported by the work of Benner (1984), who suggests that while beginning practitioners adhere to rules and procedures, the development of experience and expertise is characterised by the transcendence of rule-bound behaviour to allow more spontaneity, the exercise of discretion, and the use of what appears to be intuitive behaviour.

The New Nursing?

Whether or not it is helpful to coin terms such as 'The New Nursing' to describe what has been happening in the UK, there is no doubt that an increasingly influential group of writers over the last 30 years or so have mounted a strong challenge to the traditional view of nursing. If traditional nursing was characterised by its dependence on the medical profession, hierarchical structures, centralised decision-making, and on fragmentation of care, functional approaches to care delivery, and the denial or avoidance of the nurse–patient relationship, these are precisely the characteristics that nurse theorists and leaders of the profession have sought to change.

The first evidence of change can be traced at least as far back as the 1960s in the USA, and probably as far back as the 1950s with the work of Lydia Hall. Perhaps the most influential definition of nursing is Henderson's, and I make no apologies for quoting it again here:

'The unique function of the nurse is to assist the individual, sick or well, in the performance of those activities contributing to health or its recovery (or to a peaceful death) that he would perform unaided if he had the necessary strength, will or knowledge. And to do this in such a way as to help him gain independence as rapidly as possible. This aspect of her work, this part of her function, she initiates and controls; of this she is master'. (Henderson 1966).

Two things are particularly striking about this statement. The first is the shift of emphasis from that of the nurse as the doctor's assistant to the nurse as the assistant to the patient. This may seem at first to be no more than juggling with words, but in fact it represents a significant shift of attitude. If we start from the assumption that human development leads toward a state of (relative) independence and responsibility for one's self, we see that most people meet their own needs for health care either from their own knowledge and experience or through popular, lay wisdom. We diagnose our own minor ailments and self-medicate, or we discuss the problem with a member of the family, a friend, or the local pharmacist. We may get ideas from popular literature, but we purchase the remedy and administer it ourselves.

If the problem cannot be managed in this way we may seek professional advice, but once again we will usually accept responsibility for following that advice and administering any treatment to ourselves. We only seek help with aspects of care, as opposed to diagnosis and prescription, when we lack the capacity to care for ourselves. The function of the nurse is thus to act on behalf of the patient, doing those things that the patient is now unable to do, and becoming in a sense part of the patient.

The second striking aspect of Henderson's (1966) definition is the final assertion that 'This aspect of her work, this part of her function, she initiates and controls; of this she is master'. This suggests a dramatic change in attitudes, both on the part of the nurse in direct contact with the patient and on the part of all the other actors in health care settings. If nurses accept this position they are at the same time declaring their independence from medicine and denying the need for the elaborate bureaucratic hierarchies that have characterised nursing for so long. They would be moving away from the situation described by Menzies, of 'collusive social redistribution of responsibility', 'purposeful obscurity in the formal distribution of responsibility', and the 'reduction of impact of responsibility by delegation to superiors'. Instead nurses would be accepting direct responsibility and accountability for their actions, for the consequences, and for the decision making process that led to those actions.

One of the most important developments that has shaped new approaches to nursing is the concept of primary nursing, and this model of care delivery typifies the changes needed to move away from the traditional, dependent position of nursing. Many discussions of the implementation of primary nursing focus on structural and organisational factors such as staff allocation and off-duty rotas which enable continuity of patient allocation. More recently the government's 'named nurse' initiative has concentrated attention on the identity of the primary nurse. Indeed in many units the most outward and visible sign of the introduction of primary nursing has been the appearance of notices at the entrance to the ward and above the beds, stating the name (and colour!) of the 'team', or the names of primary and associate nurses.

Hegedus and Bourdon (1982) describe an evaluation tool for nursing practice under primary nursing, but of the examples they give of criteria the only ones which are specific to primary nursing are:

(1)   Primary Nursing Board gives name of patient and primary nurse;
(2)   Primary Nursing Board gives name of associate nurse;
(3)   primary nurse identified in record; and
(4)   can you tell me the name of your primary nurse?

Mead (1993) used a Delphi study to identify a set of attributes which were seen as important indicators of the development of primary nursing in a clinical area and to weigh these attributes in terms of their importance as discriminating features of primary nursing. Among those most heavily weighted were items such as 'Accountability, authority, responsibility for a case load of patients' and 'Decentralised decision making', while the two least heavily weighted were 'Patients know their nurse' and 'Visual evidence of a system'.

In a survey of NHS institutions in Wales, Mead (1993) found that two out of three wards showed some characteristics of primary nursing, but the characteristics found least often were those associated with devolved decision making, achieving appropriate skill mix and case load attachment from admission to discharge. There is thus a tendency for wards to display what Mead calls the trappings of primary nursing while finding it much more difficult to adopt fundamental changes affecting authority and responsibility.

One of the most important authors in the development of primary nursing, Manthey, seems to put much more emphasis on theoretical and attitudinal frameworks. She insists for example that 'decentralised decision making is the organisational theory that provides the best foundation for primary nursing', and by this she means that the authority for decision making is located at the level of action (Manthey 1980). She justifies this assertion on the basis of the nature of work in hospitals: centralised decision making is appropriate where 'the product of the functions performed is inanimate and where the tasks used to accomplish the functions are repetitive, mechanistic, automatic, and predictable'. If the product involves human beings and the tasks are not repetitious, automatic or predictable, decentralised decision making is appropriate. Specifically,

'... when the outcome of an action is unpredictable, as with any human reaction to a stimulus, control must rest at the level of action for the most efficient and economical operation. Obviously, hospitals, where the product involves human beings (where predictability is always questioned) ought to be organised around the theory of decentralised decision making' (Manthey 1980).

It could be argued that the introduction of functional or task-centred approaches to care delivery was based on an assumption (explicit or implicit) that people in hospital could be treated as if they were inanimate and the tasks could be reduced to the extent that they became 'repetitive, mechanistic, automatic, and predictable'. This certainly is suggested by Reverby's description of the introduction of 'scientific management' theories in the 1920s (Reverby 1987). Strategies that Menzies has explained from a Freudian psychoanalytical perspective in terms of the avoidance of anxiety, and Davies as a sociologist views as evidence of power structures in the division of labour, may also be seen from the perspective of factory management and production control: the search for simplicity, economy and efficiency results in the depersonalisation and the dehumanising of staff and patients.

One of Manthey's key points is that one cannot be held responsible for anything unless one has the appropriate authority to act (Manthey 1980). Thus she believes that the primary nurse should have responsibility for the care of her case load of patients, but in order to be held responsible and accountable she must also have the authority to take decisions about the nature of that care. The reductionist, functional approach seeks to reduce the level of responsibility and thus the need for authority to the minimum. The production line worker is responsible for repeating a prescribed task in a defined way and the only authority they require is the right to perform the task and the ability to respond to an emergency or obvious deviation from normal; in the past nursing work has been reduced to this level, or very nearly so.

On the other hand it need not be like that. Gray and Pratt (1989) argue that in Australia 'society grants nurses, through licensure, the right to provide health care in the expectation that nurses will honour society's trust and be accountable for the quality of the nursing services provided'. In the UK the Nurses, Midwives and Health Visitors Act 1979 defines the competencies which must be demonstrated in order for an individual's name to be added to the professional register. The Act says nothing about the authority or responsibility of the qualified practitioner to perform to this level of competence, but one would hardly think that there would be a statutory requirement that a practitioner should be able to do something if there was not an assumption that they would be expected to put it into practice. The competencies are framed in terms of assessing the needs of patients for nursing care, for planning care and for implementing and evaluating that care. It is difficult to see how one can be responsible for assessing, planning, implementing and evaluating unless one also has the necessary authority to make decisions about the delivery of care.

Conclusions

It looks as if the arguments presented in this chapter have come full circle. The discussion began with a review of the nature of professions and the division of labour between various occupational groups and I have tried to show that for many years nurses practising in direct contact with patients had little or no authority or control over their work. The position of nursing can be viewed from the perspectives of social history, psychoanalytical theory, sociological perspectives on the division of labour in organisations, or theories of management and production control. I have tried to show that essentialist approaches to the definition of professions must fail, as must attempts to find a unitary meaning for nursing itself. There is no one set of attributes that characterise nursing and which could therefore be used to define what is the role of the nurse and what might represent variation, extensions or expansions of that role.

However, the debate about what should be an appropriate task or function for a nurse to perform continues. This in itself is significant. If nursing was simply a dependent occupation, with the nurse as the doctor's obedient assistant, then surely the problem would not have arisen, or would have been tackled as a straightforward industrial dispute. None of the tasks generally considered as extensions of the role are inherently very difficult and most if not all are performed by other types of worker with far less education than nurses, as well as by many patients and their lay carers. Heart by-pass machines are operated by skilled technicians. Much of the work in the operating theatre can be done by technicians. Emergency resuscitation and life support is carried out by ambulance staff who frequently find themselves handing their patient over to 'professional' staff who are far less skilled in this area than the paramedics.

Nursing is still very much in a transitional state. On the one hand we have the development of primary nursing and arguments for autonomy and self-governance, reinforced by initiatives such as the named nurse, nurse prescribing, the development of specialist and advanced practitioners, and the reduction of junior doctors' hours. In the international arena we have a view of the nurse expressed by bodies such as the World Health Organization, which envisages something well beyond the notion of a dependent, subordinate worker (Nakajima 1992; WHO 1988).

On the other hand we have, apparently, a deep desire on the part of many nurses to be part of the team and to continue in the *status quo*. Buckenham and McGrath (1983) found that nurses in hospital wards in Australia showed a primary allegiance to the professional health care team and would only act, for example, as patient advocate if this did not jeopardise membership of that team. Nurses saw their main function as assisting and supporting the doctor, displaying a deep loyalty that seemed to be related to the desire to stay in the team, even though the price of membership was subordination.

We have through the NHS reforms the new 'managerialism', which increases the power of the general manager and the accountant over the desires of the practitioner. One hears many anecdotes that illustrate this, such as that of the general manager who cancelled an order for the hire of a specialist pressure-relieving bed required for a patient who was terminally ill and at severe risk of developing pressure sores. The rationale for cancelling the order was that since the patient was dying there was no return on the expenditure (Mead, personal communication, 1993). Two things emerge from this anecdote and others like it: one is the attitude of the individual concerned; the other is that he had the authority to cancel the order without reference to the professional who initiated it and indeed had not even informed the ward of his decision. It would seem that Keyzer (1992) is right, and in the new order the general manager does have the authority to define the scope of nursing practice.

It is unlikely that the tensions within the various occupational groups in the health care setting, both between the various professions and between professionals and managers, will ever be resolved in fixed relationships and boundaries. It is in the nature of such relationships that there will be continuing changes in the light of new priorities and shifts in the balance of power. Nursing could yet be submerged and lost in the swamp of competence-based training and vocational qualifications. Nurses could become instrumental workers, directed by doctors but managed by accountants. Nurses could seize the high moral ground of health care, working for the benefit of the patient in whatever shape or form that might take, and determining for themselves what skills are required and what tasks should be performed.

Documents such as the UKCC's *Code of Professional Conduct* (UKCC 1992a) and *The Scope of Professional Practice* (UKCC 1992b) suggest a scenario in which nurses function with some degree of professional autonomy, but until nurses can achieve the requisite authority they will not be able to realise more than a fraction of the possibilities suggested by these documents.

Nursing abounds with paradoxes. In spite of the many strategies adopted by nurses to avoid responsibility it is a common complaint that nurses feel they are expected to take responsibility for every aspect of patient care and for the smooth running of the hospital; they feel this (and there is some truth in it) in spite of manifestly not having the authority to take decisions and to have those decisions upheld and supported by others within the organisation. They adopt the trappings of primary nursing and the concept of the named nurse in spite of the inability to establish essential features such as decentralised decision making and the accountability, authority and responsibility for a case load of patients.

The UKCC's *The Scope of Professional Practice* document was a response to mounting criticisms of the DHSS position on the so-called 'extended role' (see Appendix V). The document advocates the rejection of specific task-related competencies and certification in favour of a more general individual responsibility for personal development. But it says nothing about the nurse's <u>*authority*</u> for making decisions about the scope of nursing practice, either in the sense of choosing which skills, procedures or treatments a nurse may take on, or in the sense of determining when or whether any such procedures might be appropriate for any individual patient. The real test of the development of nursing as a profession and the scope of professional practice will be the extent to which nurses do not just take on the responsibility for additional tasks, but the extent to which they achieve authority over the nature of their practice.

References

Ashdown A. M. (1943) *A Complete System of Nursing*, 2nd edn. J. M. Dent, London.

Bayles M. D. (1989) *Professional Ethics*, 2nd edn. Wadsworth, Belmont, USA.

Benner P. (1984) *From Novice to Expert: Excellence and Power in Clinical Nursing Practice*. Addison Wesley, Menlo Park, USA.

Buckenham J. E. & McGrath G. (1983) *The Social Reality of Nursing*. ADIS Health Science Press, Balgowlah.

Cleland V. S. (1975) Taft-Hartley amended: implications for nursing – the professional model. *American Journal of Nursing* **25** (2), 288–292.

Davies C. (1976) Experience of dependency and control in work: the case of nurses. *Journal of Advanced Nursing* **1**, 273–282.

Dingwall R., Rafferty A. M. & Webster C. (1988) *An Introduction to the Social History of Nursing*. Routledge, London.

Department of Health and Social Security (1977) *The extending role of the clinical nurse – legal implications and training requirements*. DHSS, London.

Department of Health and Social Security (1989) *The extending role of the nurse*. DHSS, London.

Etzioni A. (1969) *The Semi-Professions and Their Organisation.* The Free Press, New York.

Friedson E. (1970) *The Profession of Medicine.* Dodd, Mead, New York.

Gray G. & Pratt R. (1989) Accountability: pivot of professionalism. In *Issues in Australian Nursing 2* (eds G. Gray & R. Pratt). Churchill Livingstone, Melbourne.

Hegedus S. J. & Bourdon S. M. (1982) Evaluation research: a quality assurance program. In *Perspectives in Primary Nursing* (ed. B. J. Brown). Aspen, Rockville, USA.

Henderson V. (1966) *The Nature of Nursing.* Macmillan, New York.

Keyzer D. (1992) Nursing policy, the supply and demand for nurses: towards a clinical career structure for nurses. In *Policy Issues in Nursing* (eds J. Robinson, A. Gray & R. Elkan). Open University Press, Buckingham.

Kloss D. K. (1988) Demarcation in medical practice: the extended role of the nurse. *Professional Negligence* March/April 41–47.

McKee M. & Lessof L. (1992) Nurse and doctor: whose task is it anyway? In *Policy Issues in Nursing* (eds J. Robinson, A. Gray & R. Elkan). Open University Press, Buckingham.

Manthey M. (1980) A theoretical framework for primary nursing. *The Journal of Nursing Administration* **10** (6), 11–15.

Mead D. M. (1993) *The development of primary nursing in National Health Service care giving institutions in Wales.* Unpublished PhD Thesis, University of Wales.

Menzies I. (1960) A case study in the functioning of social systems as a defence against anxiety – a report on a study of the nursing services of a general hospital. *Human Relations* **13**, 95–121.

Ministry of Health, Scottish Home and Health Department (1966) *Report of the Committee on Senior Nursing Staff Structure.* HMSO, London.

Nakajima H. (1992) Editorial: more than ever, we need nurses. *World Health* Sept–Oct, 3.

Pembrey S. (1980) *The ward sister – key to nursing.* Royal College of Nursing publication, London.

Reverby S. M. (1987) *Ordered to Care: The Dilemma of American Nursing 1850–1945.* Cambridge University Press, Cambridge.

Rowbottom R. (1978) Professionals in health and social service organisations. In *Health Services* (ed. E. Jaques). Heinemann, London.

Salvage J. (1992) The new nursing: empowering patients or empowering nurses? In *Policy Issues in Nursing* (eds J. Robinson, A. Gray & R. Elkan). Open University Press, Buckingham.

Sleicher M. N. (1981) Nursing is not a profession. *Nursing and Health Care* April 186–191, 218.

Stein L. I. (1967) The doctor–nurse game. *Archives of General Psychiatry.* **16**, 699–703.

United Kingdom Central Council for Nursing, Midwifery and Health Visiting (1992a) *Code of Professional Conduct.* UKCC, London.

United Kingdom Central Council for Nursing, Midwifery and Health Visiting (1992b) *The Scope of Professional Practice.* UKCC, London.

Vollmer H. M. & Mills D. L. (1966) *Professionalisation.* Prentice Hall, Englewood Cliffs, USA.

World Health Organization (1988) *Summary Report: European Conference on Nursing.* WHO, Vienna.

Wittgenstein L. (1958) *Philosophical Investigations.* Translated by G. E. M. Anscombe. Macmillan, New York.

Chapter 2
New Professionals? New Ethics?

Introduction

To understand the significance of the professional ethics of nursing in the context of role expansion requires an understanding of the nature of professionalism and of the wider changes occurring across the whole gamut of professional life. The professionalisation of nursing is an aspect of the wider trend of the professionalisation of work in the industrial countries (Perkins 1989).

Professional groups nearly always have 'ethics', usually embodied in some code.[1] In the most general terms, the need for professional ethics arises because a profession is a group which separates itself from society at large by virtue of its expertise (or claim to expertise). This expertise endows it with power which is problematic and contestable since it can be used for good or bad. Ethics (or 'professional conduct') is the attempt to give moral homogeneity to the group's specific practices and to address the problematic relationship between that group and everyone else.

The rationale of professional codes is controversial, and is probably inherently ambivalent (Edgar 1994; Kultgen 1988). On one interpretation a code of ethics serves to close off the profession from the 'laity' and legitimise its power, that is, it protects the profession from the public (closure). On another view an ethics serves to bring together the profession and the public in mutual trust and purpose, that is, it protects the public from the profession (openness). Rather than engage in a fruitless effort to establish which of these interpretations is 'correct', it is assumed that it is in the nature of the case that professional ethics is *ambivalent* in this regard. A better understanding is gained by examining the nature of the professional ethics of nursing from both sides.

There is little doubt that many have come to see the traditional professions (such as medicine, law, pharmacy, accountancy) as promoting an ethics of closure. But the professions have undergone fundamental changes in the last two or three decades, changes which have generated pressure for a professional ethics of openness. Some professions have taken this more seriously than others; the traditional professions have tended to dig in their heels by uncritically reiterating the claim that their ethical position was always about public trust and protection whatever the critics may have said.

On the one hand, there is a continuation of a trend to specialisation and expertise and, on the other, there is a dramatic reorientation of professionalism itself under the impact of industrial management for the market. We have, then, two groups of distinctions to make in considering the significance of role expansion in nursing (see Fig. 2.1). This chapter is an exploration of what role expansion in nursing means for the possibility of a new ethics of openness, in the light of increased technical specialisation and the new managerial and commercial environment.

Closure and openness

The medical profession

The ethics of closure is associated with the traditional role of the health care professional. Looked at as an 'ideal type', this professional was a generalist in skills and knowledge and was inclined to see illness and health in a personal, family and social context. Furthermore, the traditional professional may have received a high income, but this was regarded as a reward for dedicated public service rather than for the achievements of exercising entrepreneurial skills in producing and marketing a commodity. Indeed, ideally the professional was a devoted and skilled expert who had some understanding of what was 'in the patient's best interest', exercised 'clinical judgement' and worked for the public welfare as a principal goal.

---

1 *Professionals*
(a) The traditional professional
(b) The new professional
    (i)   Increased technical specialisation
    (ii) Industrial management
    (iii) A commercial environment

2 *Ethics*
(a) Ethics of closure
(b) Ethics of openness

Fig. 2.1 Two distinctions to make when considering role expansion in nursing.

An ethics of closure was attendant on this view of the public sector professional. The burden of judgement always lay entirely with the professional. The doctor, for example, was not seen as a technician who might give advice, so much as one who really understood what was good for patients and knew what their needs were better than patients themselves did. In this understanding of things the question of openness and closure did not even arise, for patients saw no alternative to trust in the judgement of the doctor. The closure which we now see when we look back with a critical eye on past practices and attitudes was not seen as such at the time, but rather as the justified reserve, tact and wisdom of the medical profession.

The special respect which was owed to the professions rested on these perceptions. Nurses partook of this special respect, but only in so far as they were in on the doctor's act. They were in on it in the first place because nurses were taught by doctors (Keddy *et al.*, 1986). Like the patient, the nurse for the most part left the burden of judgement with the doctor. Everyone had their allotted place. Closure was so complete that openness, in the modern sense, was not even conceivable.

The General Medical Council's disciplinary procedures and its document *Professional Conduct and Discipline: Fitness to Practise* are still largely based on the assumptions of closure (GMC 1991). Thus strong concerns with 'the reputation of the medical profession' and discouraging the 'disparagement of professional colleagues' would appear to put the emphasis on protecting the profession rather than substantive issues of patients' rights and freedom.

The medical ethics of closure was already challenged by the critiques of the 1960s. The doctor is now often widely viewed with some suspicion, alternative therapies have the allegiance of thousands, and the entire medical profession has been subjected to (admittedly not always fair) accusations of paternalism, high-handedness and self-interested protectionism (Illich 1976; Kennedy 1983). We can no longer take it for granted that paternalistic professionalism is what the public wants. Certainly, it wants skill and dedication, but does it want an elite which takes 'clinical judgement' and self-regulation as an opportunity to protect its own interests, free from public scrutiny?

Nursing in general

Traditionally the nurse had the role of doctor's handmaiden, so that the question of the nurse's ethics, if it arose at all, was reduced to one of obedience. Thus the nurse was expected to respect confidences which she gleaned in the course of the doctor's treatment and examination of the patient, and above all had to cooperate with and facilitate the doctor's work. The idea of an ethics peculiar to nursing, which went beyond obedience, would have been alien in the traditional scheme of things. Indeed, nursing ethics is a recent phenomenon closely related to the increasing autonomy and professionalisation of nursing.

This leaves nursing with a question. Is it to adopt the traditional (medical) ethics of closure as it encroaches on the medical role? Alternatively, will it take as its point of departure the more personal, understanding and immediate character of nursing to develop an ethics of openness? This is where the question of the significance of role expansion and the significance of nursing ethics interlock.

In many ways the professional ethics of nursing holds out great promise, and potentially would appear to be in advance of the ethics of many other professional groups. Jean Robinson, lay member on the General Medical Council (GMC), has compared the workings of the GMC with that of the nurses' regulatory body set up in 1979, the United Kingdom Central Council (UKCC). She points out many ways in which nurses are far ahead of doctors in moving towards an ethics of openness. She is concerned about medical protectionism and writes:

'Nurses are charged with 'professional misconduct' whereas doctors can only be charged with '*serious* professional misconduct'. Why, I wonder, should the public be more effectively protected against the unsafe nurse than the unsafe doctor?... Despite its lack of lay members, the UKCC council may be doing a better job of protecting the public than the GMC.' (Robinson 1988, p. 39)

Still, there is a great disparity between, on the one hand, the move towards openness which appears in the UKCC's *Code of Professional Conduct* and in the recent improvements in its structure and procedures and, on the other, the actual economic, political and administrative background of nursing. Regulatory enhancement of the responsibility for patients and a demand for sensitivity to the needs and values of patients have not been accompanied by an increase in the real institutional freedom of nurses to judge, decide and act.

This tension in nursing between the ethics of institutional closure and of individual openness is manifest in the new (third) edition of the UKCC's *Code of Professional Conduct* (UKCC 1992b). This edition makes it clearer that the primary statutory obligation of the UKCC is not to protect the professions, but to protect the public (Hunt 1992a). However, at the same time it removes any hint of support for the view that nurses have a legitimate interest in managerial and resource matters or, to put it differently, it sharpens the divide between managerial concerns and nursing concerns. This makes it more difficult for a nurse to speak up on behalf of patients where problems are caused by poor management and resource shortages.

The Code

Let us look at the third edition of the Code in greater detail, to clarify what is meant by its promotion of openness. Greater weight is given to patients and their families. There is a welcome new emphasis on working in a cooperative and enabling spirit with patients, and on the important contribution of 'informal' carers. The old edition (UKCC 1984) had the defect that there was no explicit warning about discrimination against patients. But we now have:

> '... recognise and respect the uniqueness and dignity of each patient and client, and respond to their need for care, irrespective of their ethnic origin, religious beliefs, personal attributes, the nature of their health problems or any other factor.'

The last point is particularly important in relation to HIV/AIDS.

To the old section about not abusing privileged access to patients has been added 'to their person' as well as 'to property, residence or work-place'. This is a recognition that the professions should protect the privacy of patients, which is a wider duty than protecting information about them (confidentiality). After all, ridiculing a patient's body or allowing strangers a view of the patient's private parts menaces the trusting relationship as much as stealing the patient's wallet.

Now let us look at some detail which illustrates what is meant by the ethics of closure. There is a slightly more cautious wording on the controversial issue of the environment of care. The second edition's phrases, 'adequacy of resources' and 'the workload of and pressures on' colleagues, have been deleted. More subtly, whereas the second edition stated 'Have regard for the environment of care', it is now its effects one should have regard for.

Managers often say to concerned or dissenting nurses that resources, workload, and pressures are a managerial matter and none of their business. Dissenters, in fear of victimisation for expressing concerns, could before at least hold up the Code and say to managers, 'It is my business. It says I should have regard for the environment of care'. The third edition says instead that the nurse should report to an appropriate person or authority circumstances in the environment of care which could jeopardise standards of practice and circumstances in which safe and appropriate care for patients cannot be provided. But the word 'circumstances' is so general as to be nearly useless. And who is an 'appropriate person or authority'? One doubts that these words were intended to include, if all else fails, a Member of Parliament, a Consumer Health Council, a patients' watchdog, or a journalist.

The wider the scope of a generalisation in a code or regulation the wider the scope for disagreement about what it means and how to apply it, and the easier it is for the stronger party to make its interpretation prevail. It is possible that a manager might say to a dissenting nurse that the Code's 'circumstances' do not include economic or administrative matters, but strictly a narrow spectrum of nursing matters.

The old section 11 advised nurses 'to take appropriate action' if the workload and pressures were 'seen to be such as to constitute abuse of the individual practitioner and/or to jeopardise safe standards of practice'. 'Take appropriate action' would appear to leave some judgement to the practitioner, and quite rightly. That has been replaced with 'report to an appropriate person or authority', which is surely somewhat stale hierarchical thinking. Moreover, the word 'abuse' has gone and been replaced with 'health or safety of colleagues', and the 'and/or' has gone too.

The significance of the latter is that the 'or' implied that to justify taking action it was sufficient that a nurse was abused by their workload and pressures (even if safe standards were not consequently jeopardised). But the new section 13 says a report should be made 'where it appears that the health or safety of colleagues is at risk, as such circumstances may compromise standards of practice and care'. That is, the justification for making a report is not in itself the 'abuse' of the nurse, but rather the threat to standards of practice. However, management has enormous influence in defining what an acceptable standard of practice is, and there is evidence that this standard is being adjusted downwards while what is defined as an acceptable nursing workload is being adjusted upwards. Do these changes in the Code represent a slight retreat?

There are two sections I would like to have seen in the Code: firstly, the recognition of a duty to protect the public from misinformation and misrepresentation; secondly, a clearer recognition of a duty to establish conditions of employment conducive to excellence in nursing care. These are both embodied, for example, in the American Nurses' Association Code for Nurses (Bandman & Bandman 1990). Such clauses would address the relationshiip between the profession and management in the spirit of openness, and therefore do a great deal to strengthen all the clauses about partnership with patients.

Increased technical specialisation

Health care has seen a great degree of technical innovation and

specialisation in the last two or three decades. It has been divided
between the expertise and technology of the haematologist, the dietitian,
the podiatrist, the speech therapist, the maxillo-facial surgeon, the
oncologist, the occupational therapist, the counsellor, etc. It is not surprising that this has percolated into nursing, creating a plethora of
clinical nurse specialists such as the haematology nurse, the ICU specialist, the accident and emergency nurse, the clinical nurse specialist in
epilepsy, the stoma nurse, the neurological nurse, etc.

What does this technical specialisation mean for closure and openness? There is the danger that such a trend will work against hopes for
holistic and primary nursing. We may think about this in terms of three
aspects: fragmentation, distance and a technical mode of thought.

Fragmentation:

The fragmentation of technique tends to carry with it a corresponding
fragmentation of role and responsibilities. The danger is that it will
become increasingly difficult in many areas of care for anyone to get a
human grasp of caring for a person with health difficulties. The worst
scenario is one in which each carer is concerned with some aspect of the
patient's 'case' while no one is concerned with the patient. Clearly a
professional ethics which means nothing more than each carer completely discharging his or her obligation or duty in fulfilling narrowly
defined responsibilities is an inadequate one.

In this situation of fragmentation, which in any case should be held in
check, inter-professional liaison and multidisciplinary team-working is
an ethical prerequisite of good practice. Nurses will have to take their
own initiatives to persuade doctors to see the benefits of team working
and respect for nursing judgement (Nursing Times 1992; Hammond
1992).

The Scope of Professional Practice recognises the difficulty. It says
that the nurse, midwife or health visitor,

'...must ensure that any enlargement or adjustment of the scope of
personal professional practice must be achieved without compromising or fragmenting existing aspects of professional practice and
care and that the requirements of the Council's Code of Professional
Conduct are satisfied throughout the whole area of practice' (UKCC
1992a, section 9.4).

Indeed, the Council's rejection of role extension, as opposed to expansion, was based on anxieties about fragmentation: 'The Council also

believes that a concentration on "activities" can detract from the importance of holistic nursing care' (UKCC 1992a, section 13).

Still, it is one thing to shout at the tide, it is quite another to hold it back, as King Canute demonstrated.

Distance

Just as the medical profession's increasing control over advanced technology has distanced the patient from the doctor, resulting in a degeneration of the way the profession is regarded as a whole, so there is a danger that role expansion in nursing will have the same deleterious effect. Many specialised nurses may find themselves drawn increasingly into a biomedical role which takes them further away from patients, making it harder to understand their experience of illness or health care, and thus making it harder to *nurse*. As is pointed out in Chapter 12, it is possible that at least in the hospital setting nurses will move up an echelon in the biomedical hierarchy while health care assistants take on the traditional nursing role.

The UKCC's 'Scope' document appears to be well aware of this possibility, warning practitioners to avoid both 'inappropriate delegation to others' and, as we have seen, 'compromising' existing aspects of care (UKCC 1992a, sections 9.4, 9.6).

Technical mode of thought

There is a more insidious danger in role expansion, although I do not suggest the nursing role will necessarily develop this way. That is, many nurses will gradually come to think of themselves, their role, patients, illness and the restoration of health as a 'technical' or even 'technological' enterprise in which they are the new experts. In other words they will start to follow the same biomedical philosophy as the medical profession, with a new element of managerialism also prominent.

Regarded from a historical point of view, role expansion could turn out to be nursing's catching up rather late in the day with the process of *rationalisation* of human activity which Max Weber described (Weber 1947). In this view modern society is marked by a strong tendency to turn every human activity into a technical process which lends itself to rational analysis, explanation and 'engineering'. This trend undermines human values, replacing them with techniques. Two recent commentators have written,

'...in the nursing profession there are indications of a conflict between the process of rationalisation and fundamental values traditionally associated with the profession ... growing pressures to implement a mechanistic model in nursing tend to undermine such basic values of the nursing profession and lead to job dissatisfaction, stress, frustration and confrontation between nurses, physicians and health care administrators.' (Hewa & Hetherington 1990, p. 179)

These authors argue that the undermining of the Judaeo-Christian and vocational basis of nursing by an 'instrumental rational' attitude has resulted in a widespread crisis in nursing, and they point to North American studies which indicate widespread stress, 'burn-out', low job-satisfaction and high staff turn-over. In other words, nurses no longer feel they are doing the 'humane' and caring work which they would like to be doing. Is this what role expansion in nursing is really about? Probably what we have here is one trend, with other trends pulling in different directions.

I should also mention that one impact that increasing 'technicalisation' of care has had on the awareness that something is morally amiss is the widespread and, I think, perverse idea that ethics itself may be technicalised. Paradoxically, while technicalisation produces the moral problem of the age, technicalisation also holds out the false promise of solving it. The assumption is that moral problems are essentially technical problems, which must have technical solutions (Hunt 1994). Thus the authors of one influential bioethics text say that they 'emphasize the development of a theory and a set of principles for the treatment of [ethical] problems' (Beauchamp & Childress 1989, p. 3).

Nursing autonomy

Role expansion involves a lot more than increasing technical specialisation. It is convenient to think of the ethics of openness in terms of three other aspects of expansion: autonomy, authority and knowledge.

Autonomy

In many sectors of nursing there has over the years been an increasing degree of scope for independence of judgement, decision-making and action. However, this has been very uneven and there have been counter-trends. The idea of 'role expansion' may be seen as official sanction and support for this trend. It is not as clear what this means for the professional ethics of nursing as might at first appear.

The UKCC's Code says that practitioners are 'personally accountable' for their practice, and the 'Scope' document reiterates that they 'must recognise and honour the direct or indirect personal accountability borne for all aspects of professional practice' (UKCC 1992a, section 9.5).

For example, obtaining informed consent from the patient is as much a nurse's responsibility as that of the doctor in charge. The UKCC makes it clear that if a nurse thinks the patient has not understood a proposed examination or treatment she should seek to remedy the situation and even refuse to cooperate if convinced the patient does not understand (UKCC 1989, p. 10). Role expansion will undoubtedly put more and more of the burden for ensuring informed consent has been obtained on the shoulders of nurses. At the same time it will open the door for greater nursing responsibility for decisions about those ethically difficult cases which are common in the health care setting – the handicapped infant, the dying patient, resuscitation, the patient who refuses life-saving treatment, truth-telling and so on.

As I have already said, however, it is one thing to increase ethical responsibility and legal liability. It is another to change the institutional setting to facilitate the exercise of such responsibility. Many changes will be necessary, and some of these nurses will have to bring about themselves. At the regulatory level the GMC and UKCC may have to work more closely in future, and it is to be hoped that the UKCC will play its part in helping gradually to bring about the changes needed in the GMC which will indirectly benefit nursing care.

Authority

Given the history of nursing I think it is necessary to emphasise the way in which the freedom of nursing has always been constrained by the medical profession and more recently by management. At the same time one has to recognise the validity of the point made by Bishop and Scudder (1987) that nurses have always had a certain kind of authority:

'Of course, nurses do not have the authority to make the same decisions that physicians and administrators have, but nurses have their own particular kind of authority. Nurses have the authority and power that comes from the control of the day-to-day care of the patient.' (Bishop & Scudder 1987, p. 39)

Bishop and Scudder (1987) say that nurses do not have to enhance their authority through a struggle for 'professional autonomy' and the reform of the health care system. This is because nurses have the space to develop their existing authority by changing everyday practices in piecemeal fashion within the power relations of the *status quo*, and thus gradually bringing about policy changes. They suggest that concern with autonomy disrupts cooperative teamwork and could work against ethical practice.

No doubt the modern trend to role expansion will work in both ways. It will enhance the professional autonomy of many nurses; some will move into new managerial roles, while many others take on partial managerial functions, and even more will have authority over increasing numbers of health care assistants. (As Ashworth and Morrison note in Chapter 2, 'the focus of many experienced practitioners in clinical settings has become much more orientated towards the management of resources.') At the same time it may increase the confidence of many others and multiply the opportunities for small everyday changes.

However, increased authority means increased power for good *or for bad*. An increase in *legitimate* authority depends on partnership with, and informed control by, patients.

We live in an age in which the public is much more questioning and sceptical of authority and more aware of its rights. Nurses too need to be more aware of their employment and civil rights in asserting themselves against authorities which often act in a high-handed and unaccountable fashion. This is an aspect of 'role expansion' which is not often mentioned. I would like to think that the conscientious 'whistleblower' is the nurse who has taken the expansion of her role to its logical conclusion.

Knowledge

Nursing autonomy requires a great deal more than nurses acquainting themselves with biomedical knowledge. If nursing expansion is to be an expansion of nursing as opposed to an expansion of medicine into nursing, then nursing will need a new paradigm of what counts as health care knowledge. This is too large an issue to take on here. It will have to suffice to say that the nursing profession should help to turn the world of health care the right way up. In our upside down world the technical manipulators of the human body (doctors) have power over those who care for individuals. In a world turned the right way up those who care for individuals would have power over the mere technicians of the body.

This requires a reappraisal of what it is 'to know' something. Does the neonatologist 'know' the baby better than the mother does? Does the gerontologist 'know' my grandmother better than I do? The ethics of closure goes hand in hand with the abstruse and 'scientific' knowledge of the biomedical technocracy; the ethics of openness requires the recognition that we (the laity) already know a great deal more of what is really important than any expert could ever expropriate.

Community nursing in its various forms no doubt provides an environment more congenial perhaps to a recognition of the kind of 'knowledge' I am speaking of, and more opportunities for the development of the ethics of openness.

Nurses will need to intervene in the ethics of research and should push for representation on local research ethics committees (Hunt 1992c).

The economic environment

Industrial Management

I have mentioned the Weberian process of rationalisation. 'The development of management' is perhaps another term for the same process. Health care, and other public sectors, have recently come under an onslaught from managerial assumptions, goals and techniques. A model of health care which borrows heavily from industry, with its preoccupation with costs, throughput, efficiency, cost-effectiveness, etc., is being imposed.

Attempts to measure variables and output for the purposes of 'efficiency' have thrown up the managerial language of 'diagnosis related groupings', 'quality adjusted life years', 'quality assurance' and so on. How far will nursing be co-opted into this new public sector managerialism? How does 'role expansion' fit in?

There has already been an enormous growth of industrial-style management at the expense of nursing and medical skills and autonomy. The UK's Department of Health, responding to a question from Alan Milburn MP in 1993, admitted that between 1989 and 1991 the National Health Service lost 5850 nurses and midwives and gained 8730 managers. The administrative staff level rose by 10 530.

Business managers, who consider themselves professionals, are now dictating to doctors and nurses and propagating a new depersonalised ideology and language of health care. The social historian Harold Perkin sees this as a new form of social conflict based on:

> 'not a revival of the entrepreneurial ideal but a reaction of one part of the professional class, the private sector managers of the great corporations and their allies, who had never felt the same degree of need for state support, against the other, the public sector professionals largely employed by the state.' (Perkins 1989, p. xiv)

There occurs a 'splitting of the professional class into two warring factions' which presents us with a modern political dilemma (in which the nursing profession is caught up):

'...the unwelcome choice between the two extremes of an author-
itarian state run by powerful and domineering professional bureau-
crats and a more diffuse neo-feudal system of great private
corporations run by equally dangerous and domineering professional
managers.' (Perkins 1989, p. xiv)

The question of what nursing role expansion means, and what its
professional ethics will become, cannot ignore this 'war'. Expansion of
the nursing role involves expansion *into* the new management at the
same time that it involves an attempt to expand *away* from the new
management. Some of the new managers in the Department of Health
figures given above are nurses who have expanded their role into
management. For professional ethics this means that some nurses will
have a split allegiance: to the ethics of professional management (if
indeed there is such a thing) and the ethics of nursing. The UKCC will
increasingly be presented with difficult cases in which nurse managers
following 'industrial' goals will be at loggerheads with subordinates
defending standards of care as 'advocates' of their patients. One may
envisage increasing numbers of cases in which the subordinates attempt
to use the professional conduct required by the UKCC against their nurse
managers while the latter attempt in turn to use employment contracts
and Trust procedures against their subordinates. A war indeed.

If all nurses were to wake up one morning and start to live strictly by
the present ethical exhortations of the UKCC then one of two things
would happen: (a) The industrial management model would be set back,
or (b) The UKCC and the nursing profession would be set back.

Certainly, the question arises whether the codes and regulations of
such bodies are themselves unethical.[2] But one should not mistake a
regulatory body for a union or similar organisation. A regulatory body
behaves ethically if it attempts to do its utmost to provide and implement
the appropriate guidelines and procedures for protecting the public; but
nurses themselves have to change the general direction and political
weight of nursing. If they do not believe they can do that or think that
some other body should do it for them then it will not happen, and
nursing will remain an undercurrent in the history of other social forces.

The market and consumerism

Industrial management is complemented by the marketplace, a place in
which people appear as consumers expressing their choices by making
purchases. Illness, disease, disability and infirmity are market opportunities and health care a commodity. The displacement of health care into

the market is having, and will continue to have, wide ranging repercussions for nursing and its professional ethics (Hunt 1990, 1991, 1992b).

While the erosion of the paternalism and unfettered power of the medical establishment is welcomed by many (understandably not usually by doctors themselves), the commercialisation of health care may not be so welcome. It drives out, indeed has largely driven out, of health care what is most important in it – the idea of understanding and serving those who need help. The professional ideal in health care is in danger of being substituted by the health carer as salesman and shop assistant.

While the ethics of openness requires a partnership between health carer and patient the only kind of partnership which is workable in a commercial environment is that of the exchange contract. Here ethics is narrowed down to the proprieties of contract – a fair price, unadulterated goods, delivery on time, prompt payment and so on.

Professional health carers are finding that they can no longer always expect clinical judgement to take precedence, or even have the freedom to express concern about their patients and the standard of care they are receiving. Market demand and supply intrudes into clinical judgement. 'Whistle-blowing' has become an issue because health care professionals are finding that they cannot always sustain decent standards in the face of dwindling resources and the demands of increased 'throughput'. Whereas nurses were once able to think of themselves as people with a vocational service for which there was always a ready place in the public sector, they are now having to think in terms of nursing labour, a commodity in the free market for which there is declining demand.

Role expansion has to be seen in this context, for while some nurses specialise and upgrade their skills in order to make themselves more marketable, others have to deny their skills because in a shrinking labour market they find themselves over-qualified.

The commercial climate has a wide ranging impact on the very character of nursing. Those who work in private residential homes, private hospitals, or with budget-holding GPs and are subject to commercial pressures such as individual and local contracts of employment, sponsorship and advertising, will naturally adopt an attitude about their responsibilities which is quite different from the traditional one.

The different echelons of nursing will no doubt react to these changes in different ways. The old guard of genteel professionals typified by the traditional ward sister will be suspicious and cautious; the aggressive professionals typified by nurse management and 'high-tech' nursing will probably welcome them with open arms; and the anti-professionals typified by the pragmatic grass roots nurse may to some extent resist them.

However, on the whole commercialisation will tend gradually to undermine the very notion of professional ethics as presently understood in nursing (and other occupations) (Hunt 1992b). The UKCC may publish advice about, for example, commercial sponsorship and advertising but how long will it be before such advice is ignored or treated with lip-service? (UKCC 1985)

Conclusion

The crisis in health care provides a new opportunity for a debate about professionalism, and a new understanding of what a professional is or should be. If this opportunity is not seized then the professional will also be swallowed up by the market and will lose the traditional sense of social conscience and public service, surely worth saving, and take on the garb of the businessman or businessman's employee. Ironically, this will happen at the very time when there is a felt need for reappraisal of our understanding of business management and corporate responsibility.

Role expansion is a much wider issue than increasing the kinds of tasks nurses can properly undertake. It is about the very character of nursing itself and the possibility of a professional ethics of openness.

Will 'role expansion' mean the expansion of nursing itself, or the expansion of management, medicine and the market into nursing?

Notes

1   The term 'ethics' is used in several different ways:
    (a)   A branch of philosophy, characterised by an attempt to grasp the general nature of morality or the logic of moral discourse, e.g. the ethics of Immanuel Kant.
    (b)   Common morality, e.g. when I say 'I don't think much of his ethics'.
    (c)   A more or less coherent system of rules or principles constituting a world view or part of a world view, as in 'Christian ethics'.
    (d)   The codified moral principles intended to regulate the behaviour of a group, as in 'professional ethics'. It is the last I am concerned with.
2   Regarding the GMC, Jean Robinson writes: 'The GMC often makes pronouncements on ethical issues for the profession. But what are the ethics of the Council itself when it holds in its files serious alle-

gations which suggest the public could be at risk, which are not even seen by the Preliminary Screener? To reach him, complaints must first survive the ordeal of the NHS procedure obstacle race, in which there are comparatively few winners' (Robinson, 1988, p. 13).

References

Bandman E. & Bandman B. (1990) *Nursing Ethics Through the Lifespan.* Appleton & Lange Norwalk. The ANA Code is reprinted in the Appendix.

Beauchamp T. L. & Childress J. F. (1989) *Principles of Biomedical Ethics*, 3rd edn. Oxford University Press, New York.

Bishop A. H. & Scudder J. R. (1987) Nursing ethics in an age of controversy. *Advances in Nursing Science* **9** (3), 34–43.

Edgar A. (due for publication in 1994) The value of codes of conduct. In *Ethical Issues in Nursing* (ed. G. Hunt) Routledge, London.

General Medical Council (1991) *Professional Conduct and Discipline: Fitness to Practise.* GMC, London.

Hammond K. (1992) Breaking professional barriers. *Nursing Standard* **6** (42), 45.

Hewa S. & Hetherington R. W. (1990) Specialists without spirit: crisis in the nursing profession. *Journal of Medical Ethics* **16**, 179–184.

Hunt G. (1990) 'Patient choice' and the National Health Service review. *Journal of Social Welfare Law* **4**, 245–255.

Hunt G. (1991) *Nursing, patient choice and the NHS reforms.* National Board for Nursing, Midwifery & Health Visiting for Northern Ireland. Fourth Annual Celebrity Lecture: Occasional Paper, Belfast, October 1991.

Hunt G. (1992a) Changing the Code. *Nursing Times* **88** (25), 21–22.

Hunt G. (1992b) Project 2000 – ethics, ambivalence & ideology. In *Project 2000: The Teachers Speak* (eds O. Slevin & M. Buckenham). Campion Press, Edinburgh.

Hunt G. (1992c) Local research ethics committees and nursing: a critical look. *British Journal of Nursing* **1** (7), 349–351.

Hunt G. (1994) Introduction. In *Ethical Issues in Nursing* (ed. G. Hunt). Routledge, London.

Illich I (1976) *Limits to Medicine.* Marion Boyars, London.

Keddy B., Jones Gillis M., Jacobs P. *et al.* (1986) The doctor–nurse relationship: an historical perspective. *Journal of Advanced Nursing* **11**, 745–753.

Kennedy I. (1983) *The Unmasking of Medicine.* Paladin, London.

Kultgen J. (1988) The ideological use of professional codes. In *Ethical Issues in Professional Life* (ed. J. C. Callahan). Oxford University Press, Oxford.

Nursing Times (1992) Correspondence on primary nursing in the 'Letters' columns of vol. 88, 24 June and 22 July.

Perkins H. (1989) *The Rise of Professional Society: England Since 1880.* Routledge, London.

Robinson J. (1988) *A Patient Voice at the GMC.* Health Rights Ltd, London.

United Kingdom Central Council for Nursing, Midwifery and Health Visiting (1984) *Code of Professional Conduct for the Nurse, Midwife and Health Visitor*, 2nd edn. UKCC, London.

United Kingdom Central Council for Nursing, Midwifery and Health Visiting (1985) *Advertising by Registered Nurses, Midwives and Health Visitors.* UKCC, London.

United Kindom Central Council for Nursing, Midwifery and Health Visiting (1989) *Exercising Accountability.* UKCC, London.

United Kingdom Central Council for Nursing, Midwifery and Health Visiting (1992a) *The Scope of Professional Practice.* UKCC, London.

United Kingdom Central Council for Nursing, Midwifery and Health Visiting (1992b) *Code of Professional Conduct for the Nurse, Midwife and Health Visitor*, 3rd edn. UKCC, London.

Weber M. (1947) *The Theory of Social and Economic Organisation*, translated by A. R. Henderson. Oxford University Press, New York.

Chapter 3
The Notion of Competence in Nursing

Introduction

✕ The expanded role of the nurse entails the exercise of additional technical expertise. The danger is that this signals a tendency to prioritise technical skills over those key personal skills and qualities which have always been central to the nursing role but which are much more difficult to practise, hard to assess and typically undervalued.

The expansion of the role of the nurse is being introduced at the same time as the 'competence' model is achieving wide acceptance in nurse education. It will undoubtedly be through competence-based education and training that the necessary new nursing skills will be developed. Again, the competence model (which describes the nursing role in terms of discrete, assessable elements of behaviour) is strongest in dealing with technical skills; it is particularly weak when it comes to those skills and qualities needed in maturely, reflectively and expertly dealing with patients and their problems (Ashworth & Morrison 1991, Ashworth & Saxton 1990).

In this chapter we show that the competence approach to education and training leads to a serious over-concern with technical aspects of the nurse's role to the great detriment of those interpersonal and personal skills and qualities which have always underlain high quality nursing practice. Personal qualities of maturity and teamwork, and skills of flexibility and wide awareness in thinking are tremendously difficult to engender. They are equally difficult to apply successfully in everyday nursing. Nursing as a profession should be far more wary of accepting a diminution in the esteem given to those skills which are most essential to good nursing practice.

Expansion of the nurse role

The expansion of the nursing role so as to embrace some further aspects of prescribing, treatment, referral and so on, has generally been welcomed. It is even arguable that there is scope for expansion beyond the boundaries currently envisaged. It seems strange to place artificial and inconsistent limits on the scope of the nurse's permitted role. Among other things, it tends to make the nurse unnecessarily dependent on medical practitioners, often in areas where it is by no means clear who has the greater expertise. Restriction in the role of the nurse can mean that in the course of dealing with the needs of the patient the nurse has to stop short, embarrassingly but routinely, in following the logic of the case and refer to 'higher authority'. Plainly the roles of the various professionals within the health care team need rational demarcation, attuned to the effective and sensitive care of the patient, rather than being based on the claims of hierarchical status and power.

The role of the nurse has changed in several important ways. There has been a noticeable tendency for the nurse to expand her role by assuming responsibility for many aspects of patients' management which have been handed down by medical colleagues. She has for example assumed responsibility for: the administration of intravenous drug therapy; male catheterisation; suturing; defibrillation; the administration of Entonox for patients in acute pain; intubation of babies; and the management of cases and teams in some community settings. In addition, the focus of many experienced practitioners in clinical settings has become much more orientated towards the management of resources.

However, it appears that there has been inadequate debate and that there is something troubling about the way in which the profession is accepting the new tasks which nurses are now being asked to include in their role. One could almost describe the attitude of many members of the profession as one of excitement and joy. This excitement is perhaps inappropriate to how the actual situation ought to be viewed – a sensible and overdue rationalisation, but nothing more.

Maybe something more is being seen in the expanded role of the nurse. It is likely that the extra element is to be found in the kind of extension envisaged: it is predominantly an expansion of *technical* skill. The role of the nurse is seen to be becoming more and more technical in its orientation. Since technical expertise is currently of higher status in our society nurses tend to view the expansion of the sphere of the profession in this direction as an advance. But is it?

The focus of nursing should surely be on holistic patient care. Technical expertise is necessary for this, of course, but the role of the nurse is centrally one which emphasises certain personal skills and qualities of patient care. Insofar as the expanded role of the nurse entails the exercise of additional technical expertise we fear that this signals an even more explicit prioritising by nurses and their managers of *technical* skills, as opposed to those key *personal skills and qualities* which are actually the central elements of the nurse's role.

The competence model in education and training

At the same time that the expansion of the nurses' role has emerged as a possibility, nurse training has begun to use as a guiding framework the notion of 'competence'. This model is one which has been developed in the UK by the National Council for Vocational Qualifications (NCVQ) and the Training Enterprise and Education Directorate of the Department of Employment (TEED, formerly known as the Training Agency, and before that, the Manpower Services Commission). The official NCVQ and TEED definition of competence-based education and training is as follows:

'... [Standards] will form the prime focus of training and the basis of vocational qualifications. Standards development should be based on the notion of competence which is defined as the ability to perform the activities within an occupation. Competence is a wide concept which embodies the ability to transfer skills and knowledge to new situations within the occupational area. It encompasses organisation and planning of work, innovation and coping with non-routine activities. It includes those qualities of personal effectiveness that are required in the workplace to deal with workers, managers and customer.'

(TEED 1988).

This notion of 'competence', which stresses the careful definition and assessment of distinct items of work performance, has been adopted as the linchpin of the new vocational qualifications system. The idea is that qualifications will be defined in terms of the specific skills, capabilities, applicable pieces of knowledge and understanding which the individual is certified as having. It is intended that these certified capacities will be closely related to job demands so that employers will know what they can expect of the people holding a recognised National Vocational Qualification (NVQ).

The Nurses, Midwives and Health Visitor Rules Approval Order (Department of Health 1983) identified nine general competencies as requirements for registration as a nurse. These specify that the nurse must be able to:

(1) advise on the promotion of health and the prevention of illness;
(2) recognise situations that may be detrimental to the health and well-being of the individual;

(3)   carry out those activities involved when conducting the comprehensive assessment of a person's nursing requirements;

(4)   recognise the significance of the observations made and use these to develop an initial nursing assessment;

(5)   devise a plan of nursing care based on the assessment with the cooperation of the patient, to the extent that this is possible, taking into account the medical prescription;

(6)   implement the planned programme of nursing care and where appropriate teach and co-ordinate other members of the caring team who may be responsible for implementing specific aspects of the nursing care;

(7)   review the effectiveness of the nursing care provided, and where appropriate, initiate any action that may be required;

(8)   work in a team with other nurses, and with medical and para-medical staff and social workers;

(9)   undertake the management of the care of a group of patients over a period of time and organise the appropriate support services.

This gives a flavour of the way in which competencies are discussed. But when specified more directly for the purposes of certifying a person as adequately trained for a particular job, the definitions become much more detailed, ending up in a lengthy set of 'Is able to...' statements for each element of the job. The competence approach is receiving central encouragement. For instance, the current Code of Professional Conduct (1984) states that nurses shall 'Take every reasonable opportunity to maintain and improve professional knowledge and competence' (Statement 3). Statements 4 and 12 also explicitly refer to competence.

It may be, however, that these statements are not using the term competence in a technical sense, and therefore do not entail acceptance of any specific model of competence (such as that of NCVQ and TEED). If so, there are plenty of other official documents which definitely do use the term technically. For instance, the ENB Framework for Continuing Professional Education (Rogers 1991), refers to Statement 3 of the Code of Conduct mentioned above, and goes on to quote with approval the recommendation of the Post-Registration Education and Practice Project (PREPP) Report (UKCC 1990): '...all nurses, midwives and health visitors should demonstrate that they have maintained and developed their professional knowledge and competence' (p. 38).

Both the ENB Framework and the PREPP study on which it is based use the competence model discussed here. The PREPP study is explicit about this, referring to competencies as we see them in seven separate important paragraphs. The Framework is more coy about the use of the word, but plainly embodies the same philosophy, couched in terms of '10 key characteristics which represent the key areas of skill, knowledge and expertise which all practitioners must have to provide the quality of care required' (Rogers 1991, p. 12).

From these and other documents it is plain that there is indeed central encouragement for the use of the competence approach to nurse education. The task of educational establishments in nursing, then, is to provide courses which will enable the learner to achieve these essential competencies (McCloskey 1981). Many institutions are beginning to design their courses around these competencies (Vaughan 1990; Ellis 1988; Whittington & Boore 1988). This approach to teaching and training as it might apply to nursing seems perfectly logical and appropriate.

However, the notion of competence cannot be the main basis of training. In particular we wish to discuss four limitations of the competence model in connection with its application to nursing.

(1) *Theoretical knowledge and understanding* is essential to being a competent nurse. But scant attention is paid to this in the way competencies are specified in the NCVQ/TEED model. Nor is it made evident in the documents mentioned above (such as the Nurses, Midwives and Health Visitor Rules Approval Order) that the 'competencies' are inadequate unless exercised with thought, wide-ranging awareness and understanding.

(2) *Maturity* is a notion which covers, in a rough-and-ready way, a number of the central personal and inter-personal skills and qualities which a nurse must have in order to engage in holistic patient care with any success. But the kind of qualities denoted by 'maturity' are not open to definition or assessment within the competence model.

(3) Being a competent nurse involves the ability to engage fully in *teamwork*. As we saw above, the nurse must 'work in a team with other nurses, and with medical and paramedical staff and social workers'. The competence movement has rightly emphasised teamwork, but it actually adopts an individualistic orientation by emphasising the personal 'ownership' of competencies.

(4) Competencies, in the TEED/NCVQ model, are defined within a strictly *behavioural analysis*, referring always to activities which the individual can perform. While this looks superficially attractive from the point of view of enabling the nurses' skills and capacities to be 'objectively' assessed, it does not in fact solve assessment problems, and additionally supports the biases mentioned above, being individualistic and failing to cover the range of relevant mental activity.

It can be argued that there is a worrying over-emphasis on technical expertise rather than holistic patient care in the competence notion, which reinforces a similar tendency in the extension of the role of the nurse.

Critique of the competence model in nursing

Theoretical knowledge and understanding

The history of the notion of competence within NCVQ and TEED indicates major uncertainty concerning the role of knowledge, and the necessity or otherwise of reflective thinking. The role of knowledge and understanding is still treated (despite a certain amount of agonizing, see Black & Wolf 1990; Fender & Stuart 1990; Jessup 1991; and Wolf 1989) in a paltry way by the advocates of the competence model. 'An element of competence may describe such things as the knowledge or understanding which is essential if performance is to be sustained, or extended to new situations within the occupation' according to the official TEED guidelines (1988). So knowledge and understanding has a limited function – keeping things going and helping transfer of skill.

This is such a travesty that it seems justifiable to spend some time spelling out exactly what 'understanding' is, and why it is almost always an essential aspect of competence, and thereby underline the point that any notion of competencies which does not give understanding a special place is lacking in credibility or construct validity. This will become clear from the following examples.

Consider two learners who can state correctly the rate, in drops per minute, that an intravenous infusion should run, so that it is administered safely over a prescribed time. The mental processes by which this is done may be very different. One learner may answer by rote, while another may have an understanding of the formula for doing these sorts of calculations, and can easily adapt this formula to calculate the infusion rate when the volume of fluid, or the type of giving set, or the time is altered. The consequences of not *understanding* exactly how the formula works may be serious for the patient or client who needs the intravenous fluid. Errors may be made through the application of the wrong formula, or worse, a nurse who does not fully understand the formula may try to bluff their way through in order to save face with their colleagues.

It is obvious that the mental activity which goes with a given nursing competence may be responsible for a later error, or a later difficulty in grasping new skills. If a competence is the outcome of behaviour, not a mental skill, then things which are central to teaching are lost. But more than this, levels of awareness of situations differ enormously, and the wider the knowledge and understanding of nurses, the better will be their ability to cope flexibly and effectively with new and challenging situations.

When people do *understand* they have at their disposal a mental representation of the situation with which they are confronted. Persons who understand can give an account to themselves of the situation, and can bring to bear on it a wide range of perspectives (see Benner 1984). The more dimensions of the situation and surrounding circumstances the person can bring into consideration, the more understanding they have. This means, among other things, that a person is able to work creatively and imaginatively.

So theoretical and other forms of knowledge can be seen as an 'interpretive resource' for the person, which enriches the account they can give of the current situation and links it to new situations which are in some ways parallel, or similar in the type of thinking which can be brought to bear on them. The mental representation of the situation, and the different realms of knowledge that can be called up, enable the person to do such things as vary the situation imaginatively so as to construe alternative possibilities ('What if I did such-and-such...', 'I wonder if this problem can be solved in a similar way to...').

Take the very simple example of the avoidance of cross-infection. A student nurse may learn what to do and what not to do by assimilating a long list of rules such as hand washing, disposal of soiled linen, bed spacing, room ventilation and so on. But this does not ensure that they know the principles involved. All of the elements need to be seen as together constituting a common theme if competent care is to be promoted. An understanding of these principles, which is guided by research findings, will allow the nurse to identify the specific types of actions which are needed to avoid cross-infection. This understanding can be applied successfully when particular patients, infectious conditions or diseases or environmental considerations present themselves. The competent nurse will be able to adapt to the particular situation through her understanding of the underlying principles.

In fact, the model of competence being advocated widely in the UK contrasts sharply with that advocated in the USA by Benner (1984) and others. On the issue of 'elements of competence' she writes:

'This approach differs from listing the elemental or enabling skills that educators teach students in their early educational experiences. In contrast, the exemplars [provided in her book] will illustrate nursing performance that represents a complex of enabling skills. Only as we see the whole can we adequately appreciate the significance of the nurse's contribution to patient welfare.' (Benner 1984, p. 41)

It is impossible, in the nature of things, to be able to predict what aspects of a situation will be central to the understanding which is needed to solve a particular problem, or to gain an appreciation of a certain key aspect of the situation. Therefore, the wider the knowledge surrounding a situation, the greater the probability that nurses will have at their disposal the relevant dimensions, or maybe find themselves able to construct, on the basis of knowledge and logic, a view of the situation which is genuinely new and will increase nursing effectiveness.

Competence in the doing of something is the only kind of competence which has been focused on by TEED and NCQV thus far. No consideration is given to a person's command of a mental representation of the field within which that kind of competence is deployed. Theoretical understanding is nevertheless crucial for enabling the nurse to function effectively.

Maturity as a 'competence'?

The notion of competence includes all 'qualities of personal effectiveness that are required in the workplace' (TEED 1988). This is a very diverse set of qualities indeed: attitudes, motives, personal interests of all kinds, perceptiveness, receptivity, openness, creativity, social skills, interpersonal maturity, aspects of personal identity, as well as knowledge, understanding, actions, and skills.

Considering the range and complexity of these qualities, is it sensible to label all these different kinds of skills and personal qualities as competencies? To what extent will it facilitate learning which will influence nursing practice? Is this a sound move educationally? Quite apart from the difficulty of specifying personal relationships in terms of competence, we fear that the perception of interpersonal skills, for instance, as simply one more kind of competence to be added to the rest, will undermine the attempt to promote genuinely patient-centred care. After carrying out other tasks, the task of relating must be fulfilled! Of course, the desirable approach would be one which viewed human relatedness as part and parcel of the whole process, not a separate task.

Many practising nurses themselves recognise the potential for a closer liaison between the basic care aspects and psychological aspects of the caring role at work. In a recent study, Morrison (1992), noted how nursing informants perceived the importance of basic care skills as a 'bridge' to developing closer psychological relationships with their patients. However, it is widely acknowledged that such basic care is often completed by the least skilled and untrained nurses and generally devalued by trained nurses and medical staff (Evers 1986). The expansion of the role of the nurse into more technical domains is likely to promote a similar form of alienation for nurses and patients.

It is worth re-emphasising that we regard the kind of personal skills and qualities represented by the idea of maturity as absolutely central to the nursing role. Yet, when it comes to relating the dimensions of maturity to competence, and trying to specify competencies which would embody these ideas, it is well-nigh impossible. Consider the various aspects of maturity laid out by Knowles (1970), who makes a brief but very rich attempt to describe their essential features (adapted in Fig. 3.1).

Teamwork and the individualistic focus

Typically, the outcomes of nursing practice are due to the work of a *group* of nurses. No specific individual's mental powers or personal skills have to be the source of a successful outcome, nor does any aspect of good nursing care have to be traceable to an individual. Teamwork is an essential feature of caring in nursing practice. Nurses work in teams to plan and do their daily work, and nurses are also members of other teams along with doctors and the paramedical professions. All of these contribute to the recovery of the individual patient.

Competencies are supposed to directly relate to work roles. They are

	From	Towards
(1)	Dependence	Autonomy
(2)	Passivity	Activity
(3)	Subjectivity	Taking account of the views of other people
(4)	Ignorance	Broad awareness
(5)	Small abilities	Extended capacities
(6)	Few responsibilities	Many responsibilities
(7)	Narrow interests	Broad interests
(8)	Selfishness	Considering the general good
(9)	Self-rejection	Self-acceptance
(10)	Amorphous self-identity	Clarity of self in work role
(11)	Focus on particulars	Focus on principles
(12)	Superficial concerns	Non-petty stance
(13)	Imitative	Original
(14)	Need for certainty	Tolerance for ambiguity
(15)	Impulsiveness	Rationality

Fig. 3.1 Meanings of maturation (after Knowles 1970).

defined on the basis of an analysis of what it is that a person has to have in order to perform a specific work function, and then detailing these capacities in terms of competencies. However, there is a serious oversight inherent in the process, because the idea of a competence assumes that it is an individual person's property, so to speak: an individual has the competence which will be certified in an NVQ, and which will enable them to perform the relevant aspect of a job. So the whole way of thinking is focused on the individual. This ignores the truly collective aspects of teamwork.

Take a management team, for instance. Belbin (1981) has shown that what is required of the team is a set of complementary skills, a group of people whose psychological types gel creatively and emotionally. No one person can have all the characteristics required: indeed some of the characteristics could not co-exist within the same skin. And if the wrong set of people are chosen for the team, it will not work. No solution to this problem is possible if one merely thinks in terms of the individuals and their separate competencies. It seems very plausible that exactly the same phenomena discovered by Belbin would be true of nursing teams, and the other teams in which nurses participate (although to our knowledge the research has not been done to show this).

Take a staff nurse who personally communicates well with a diverse range of people, while another staff nurse conveys information effectively to the relevant people by delegating this task to someone else. If competence is a personal quality, as the TEED/NVQ model asserts, only the first is competent. But in practical reality, through teamwork, the task of communication is carried out adequately in both cases. The focus here clearly should be on the overall success of the team. The competence of the team, over and above the individuals within it, is just not open to consideration using the TEED definition.

On a separate level, the fact that a particular person is adjudged to be a good member of a work group and has 'interpersonal competence' is likely to be a function of the skills of other members of the group at least as much as those of that individual, who is fortunate enough to be a member of a compatible team. The notion of competence is individualistic, and cannot deal with the performance of a nursing team, or individual performance when it is intrinsic to teamwork.

The behavioural analysis

Competencies are defined on the basis of a strictly behavioural analysis, meaning that only the activities of the nurse are taken into account, and no attention is paid to mental states and processes underlying such activities. While this looks attractive from the point of view of assessment, it brings insurmountable problems in its wake. In particular, it supports the biases mentioned above, being individualistic, and failing to cover the range of relevant mental activity, so that understanding and knowledge, and personal maturity are left out. There are however, one or two other difficulties with the notion of competence in this context, particularly claims concerning transferability and assessment.

Transferability of competencies from one context to another

NCVQ lays great emphasis on skill transfer, yet, according to the Further Education Unit (FEU), 'so far there has been no significant evidence that these intentions have been realised'. Some of the complexities involved in skill transfer are recognised by the FEU (1986):

> 'The teaching and learning strategies associated with transfer are concerned with raising the awareness of the learner with respect to his/her own learning styles and potential for transfer. The act of transfer also requires skills... These are usually related to the individual being able to identify his/her needs in a new situation, adjust or reorganise previous learning, and assess his/her performance.'

The insistence that assessment of competence should ideally occur in the workplace acknowledges the issue of transfer. It is true, for instance, that learning does not always readily transfer from the classroom to the ward. But the reason for lack of transfer is often to be seen in the shallowness of the learning – the lack of genuine understanding which takes place. And there is no guarantee that the use of competence strategies will increase the depth of understanding which accompanies learning.

Saljo (1982) insists that learning is necessarily related to the specific context in which it takes place. Thus, an individual is likely to have specifically to learn to apply academic knowledge to the work environment, and to apply knowledge gained in one work context to a novel situation. It is true that some individuals seem more readily able to see relevant applications in new contexts than others or to apply the findings of research effectively. Why this is so is, frankly, not yet really known. What can be said is that the use of competence statements to describe learning attainments does not actually address the issue of transfer at all.

Part of our scepticism about transfer goes along with an anxiety about what can be called the atomism of competence statements, which is a further aspect of the behaviouristic basis of the notion. Our view is that being able to communicate is not a free-standing competence, but relates to the thing which is being communicated and the people being communicated with.

Assessing competencies

Among other issues connected with assessment, the question of objectivity gives cause for concern. The fact that comparatively clear statements of outcome are laid down as assessment criteria in the competence model, has beguiled some into thinking that they are now in possession of a thoroughly reliable and valid assessment scheme. This is a serious misunderstanding.

Logically, prior to any question of the reliability and validity of an assessment instrument is the question of the human and social process of assessing. Assessing involves the perception of evidence about a candidate's performance by an assessor, and the formulation of a decision concerning the level of performance of the person being assessed. This is a series of events in which there is enormous, unavoidable scope for subjectivity, especially when the competencies being assessed are relatively intangible ones to do with social and personal skills, or ones in which the individual's performance is intimately connected with the context (Ashworth & Saxton 1992). Whether a person's actions will be seen as showing initiative, pushiness, or uppishness will depend largely on the person's relationship with the assessor, or on the context. The specification of assessment criteria in competence terms is unlikely to affect the degree of subjectivity in assessment one jot.

Conclusion

Of all the issues confronting nurse educators at the moment it is arguable that getting a full, critical grasp of the competence model is of greatest long-term importance. The National Vocational Qualifications movement is not going to disappear (there is no political opposition to it), and it is currently set to develop in the direction of higher education and education for the professions (NCVQ 1989). The competence model, about which we have such grave doubts, is the linchpin of this movement.

The TEED/NCVQ model of competence provides 'solutions' to the specification of learning outcomes which are inappropriate to the description of human action, or to the facilitation of the education of human beings. The more human the action, the more inappropriate the current competency model of human action is, and the more likely it is that the action will require maturity in personal skills and qualities, creative thought and understanding, and involve a team rather than the activity of an individual alone. If this is true generally, it is emphatically the case as far as nurse education and training is concerned.

We are convinced that the core of nursing is precisely to do with such things as interpersonal skills and personal maturity, teamwork and the flexible application of wide-ranging knowledge – all of which finds competence an inadequate model. The expanded role of the nurse entails the exercise of additional technical expertise and, given the current situation in nurse training, it is certain that the competence model will be applied in equipping the nurse to take on the required expansion of skills.

These two trends, the adoption of competence-based education and training and the expansion of the nurse's role come together in giving even more explicit priority to technical skills as opposed to those key personal skills and qualities which we have asserted to be central to nursing. Such skills are immensely difficult to foster and to apply consistently in everyday nursing. The profession should certainly not accept unreflectively, either through extending the role of the nurse, or through adopting a competence model of training and education, a further de-emphasis of those skills which are actually most central to nursing.

In a recent publication, the UKCC (1992b) sets out its perspective on the scope of professional practice as the role of the nurse, midwife and health visitor has evolved and is still evolving. The Council does not favour the popular approach to role development which has so far emphasised the collection of a series of 'certificates' which espouse the holder's specialist technical competence. Instead the Council favours replacing such an approach with a set of principles, such as serving the interests of the client, developing professional skills and knowledge, and exercising personal accountability, which may 'provide a realistic, effective and rational approach to adjustments to professional practice' (UKCC 1992b, p.12). Moreover, the Council also rejects the use of the terms 'extended' or 'extending' role since they are seen to 'limit, rather than extend, the parameters of practice. As a result, many practitioners have been prevented from fulfilling their potential for the benefit of patients' (UKCC 1992b, p. 7). The approach recommended by the UKCC presents nurse teachers with an opportunity for reflecting critically on the competence model of training.

References

Ashworth P. D. & Morrison P. (1991) Some problems of competence-based nurse education. *Nurse Education Today* 11, 256–260.

Ashworth P. D. & Saxton J. (1990) On 'competence'. *Journal of Further and Higher Education* **14** (2), 3–25.

Ashworth P. D. & Saxton J. (1992) *Managing Work Experience.* Routledge, London.

Belbin R. M. (1981) *Management Teams: Why they Succeed or Fail.* Heinemann, London.

Benner P. (1984) *From Novice to Expert: Excellence and Power in Clinical Nursing Practice.* Addison-Wesley, Menlo Park,California.

Black H. & Wolf A. (1990) *Knowledge and Competence,* Careers and Occupational Information Centre/HMSO, London.

Department of Health (1983) *The Nurses, Midwives and Health Visitors Rules Approval Order.* HMSO, London.

Ellis R. (1988) *Professional Competence and Quality Assurance in the Caring Professions.* Chapman and Hall, London.

Evers H. K. (1986) Care of the elderly sick in the UK. In *Nursing Elderly People* (ed. S. J. Redfern), pp. 293–310. Churchill Livingstone, Edinburgh.

Fender M. & Stuart D. (1990) Linking knowledge assessment to competent performance. *Competence and Assessment* **14**, 3–5.

Further Education Unit (1986) *Assessment, Quality and Competence: Staff training issues for NCVQ.* FEU, London.

Jessup G. (1991) *Outcomes: NVQs and the emerging model of education and training.* Falmer Press, Lewes.

Knowles M. S. (1970) *The Modern Practice of Adult Education: Andragogy versus Pedagogy.* Association Press, New York.

McCloskey J. C. (1981) The effects of nursing education on job effectiveness: an overview of the literature. *Research in Nursing and Health* **4**, 355–373.

Morrison P. (1992) *Professional Caring in Practice: A Psychological Analysis.* Avebury, Aldershot.

National Council for Vocational Qualifications (1989) *Extension of the NVQ framework above level iv: a consultative document.* NCVQ, London.

Rogers J. (1991) *Framework for Continuing Professional Education for Nurses, Midwives and Health Visitors: Guide to implementation.* English National Board for Nursing, Midwifery and Health Visiting, London.

Saljo R. (1982) Learning and understanding: a study of differences in constructing meaning from a text. *Goteborg Studies in Educational Sciences* **14**. Acta Universitatis Gothoburgensis, Gothenburg.

Training Enterprise and Education Directorate (1988) *Development of Assessable Standards for National Certification. Guidance Notes 1–6.* TEED, Department of Employment, Sheffield.

United Kingdom Central Council for Nursing, Midwifery and Health Visiting (1990) *The Report of the Post-Registration Education and Practice Project.* UKCC, London.

United Kingdom Central Council for Nursing, Midwifery and Health Visiting (1992a) *Code of Professional Conduct for the Nurse, Midwife and Health Visitor,* 3rd edn. UKCC, London.

United Kingdom Central Council for Nursing, Midwifery and Health Visiting (1992b) *The Scope of Professional Practice.* UKCC, London.

Vaughan B. (1990) Writing for competencies. In *Open and Distance Learning for Nurses* (ed. K. Robinson). Longman, London.

Whittington D. & Boore J. (1988) Competence in nursing. In *Professional Competence and Quality Assurance in The Caring Professions* (ed. R. Ellis). Chapman and Hall, London.

Wolf A. (1989) Can knowledge and competence mix? In *Competency Based Education and Training* (ed. J. W. Burke). Falmer Press, Lewes.

Chapter 4
Legal Aspects of Role Expansion

Introduction

This chapter begins by considering the legal significance of the concept of the extended role of the nurse, and then goes on to analyse the implications of the scope of professional practice for the professional liability of the practitioner and its likely long-term influence on nursing and midwifery.

The nurse as a doctor's handmaiden

From the legal perspective the concept of the extended role of the nurse derived from a clear perception of what the doctor did and what the nurse did. Tasks which were normally performed by doctors but which were delegated to nurses were known as 'extended role' tasks. Interestingly, the concept was not applied to the carrying out by the nurse of the work of other professions such as physiotherapists or occupational therapists, or groups of health workers such as cleaners, caterers, porters and receptionists, even though the nurse might carry out such tasks. The traditional view of the nurse's role has been very much that of the handmaiden of the doctor.

Ruling in the case of *RCN* v. *DHSS*

The House of Lords clearly reflected this attitude in the case of the *Royal College of Nursing* v. *Department of Health and Social Security* which was concerned with the nurse's role in caring for the patient during the administration of prostaglandin-induced abortions.[1] The RCN had argued that the fact that the nurse was responsible for the patient during this treatment constituted a breach of the Abortion Act which required a registered medical officer to carry out an abortion. The RCN lost in the House of Lords by a majority verdict and Lord Diplock spelt out the relationship between doctor and nurse in the situation:

'In the context of the Act what was required was that a registered medical practitioner – a doctor – should accept responsibility for all stages of the treatment for the termination of the pregnancy. The particular method to be used should be decided by the doctor in charge of that treatment; he should carry out any physical acts, forming part of the treatment, that in accordance with accepted medical practice were done only by qualified medical practitioners, and should give specific instructions as to the carrying out of such parts of the treatment as in accordance with accepted medical practice were carried out by nurses or other hospital staff without medical qualifications. To each of them the doctor or his substitute should be available to be consulted or called in for assistance from beginning to end of the treatment. In other words, the doctor need not do everything with his own hands; the section's requirements were satisfied when the treatment was one prescribed by a registered medical practitioner carried out in accordance with his directions and of which he remained in charge throughout.'

DHSS advice in 1977

Advice by the then Department of Health and Social Security on the extended role of the nurse, given in 1977, illustrates this concept of the delegated task (DHSS 1977). There are certain tasks which are primarily to be carried out by medical staff and others carried out by nurses, and if the former are given to the nurse to perform then they should be carried out only when the following conditions are present:

(1) The nurse has been specifically and adequately trained for the performance of the new task and she agrees to undertake it.
(2) This training has been recognised as satisfactory by the employing authority.
(3) The new task has been recognised by the professions and by the employing authority as a task which may be properly delegated to a nurse.
(4) The delegating doctor has been assured of the competence of the individual nurse concerned.

DHSS Advice in 1989

In 1986 a working party was set up by the Standing Medical Advisory Committee and the Standing Nursing and Midwifery Advisory Committee to review the extended role of the nurse. Its report was circulated under cover of a DHSS letter from the Chief Nursing Officer dated 26 September 1989 (DHSS 1989) (Appendix V in this volume). It considered that the principles established in 1977 remained essentially sound but they needed to be re-interpreted and re-expressed in the light of the developments in clinical practice and changes in health service organisation. They preferred the use of the word 'activities' to that of 'tasks'. The activities of the nurse were seen as falling into three categories:

(1)   activities covered by pre-registration training;
(2)   specialist activities covered by post-registration training; and
(3)   activities normally undertaken by doctors but which may be delegated in appropriate circumstances, and which may be performed by nurses with appropriate training and competence.

The working party supported the requirement that the professions should recognise a task as being appropriate as an extended role activity but did not wish to have a national list of such activities, preferring agreement to be obtained from the medical and nursing professions locally. It considered it essential that there should be approval by the local health authority, which would be liable in law, and it recommended local procedures being set up for agreement on which activities were seen as appropriate for delegation:

'These procedures will ensure that policies for the delegation of activities are rooted in a practical understanding of the clinical tasks that need to be performed, are agreed between the professions at District level, are approved by the employing authority, and are promulgated and properly understood.'

The working party emphasised the importance of the nurse being both trained and competent. It recommended that where there were approved National Board courses these should be recognised as evidence of adequate training by individual health authorities, but other local training courses may be appropriate for other activities. In addition there might be a need for individual training to be provided within the relevant clinical environment.

The working party considered it essential that there was an assessment of competence carried out on the nurse in each new clinical environment and that the clinical nurse to whom the nurse in question is accountable should be responsible for carrying out the assessment. Once the nurse is assessed as competent this should be recorded in their personal file and a written note of it made readily available on their ward or clinical department.

It also emphasised that the nurse's consent to undertake the delegated activity remained essential. If the nurse was asked before being appointed to a post, any agreement should be recorded in the letter of appointment. It was stressed that a nurse's primary commitment was to the performance of activities that fall within the customary role.

As far as second level nurses were concerned the working party accepted that it may be appropriate in certain circumstances for enrolled nurses to undertake extended role activities, but it would not be in accordance with the Statutory Instrument to give approval to direct delegation from doctors to second level nurses.

If these policies were followed legal advice suggested that the health authority would indemnify the nurse for delegated activities carried out in the course of employment.

The value of the DHSS guidance set out above was that if a nurse followed the advice and carried out the task competently then:

(1) The nurse was protected from any disciplinary action by the employer even though the work was outside the normal course of employment, since the employer had given approval to the nurse undertaking that role.

(2) The nurse was also protected against any potential professional conduct proceedings by the UKCC since that body had agreed that that was a suitable task for a nurse provided the required training had been received.

(3) The nurse was protected from any challenge by the medical staff since the task had been personally delegated to that nurse.

If, however, the nurse was delegated an appropriate task and then carried it out negligently, there would be the possibility of facing hearings in the civil courts, before the professional conduct committee, and before the employer, but the fact that it was an extended role task would not be used against the nurse. Rather it should help since the nurse was more likely to have required closer supervision in order for it to have been carried out competently.

A further advantage of the DHSS guidance was that it offered nurses a choice. If an extended role task was not considered to be part of basic nursing, even if additional training had been given, nurses could in theory refuse to undertake it if the pressure on resources was such that they did not have the time for additional duties. Thus there were cases where nurses trained to carry out the extended role task of adding drugs to intravenous drips refused instructions from junior doctors to do this work on the grounds that they were too busy. This produced a minefield of controversy and dispute, and increasingly the possibility of the nurse refusing to undertake the task disappeared. If the nurse was trained and competent then there was an expectation that the nurse would perform the task when requested.

Increasingly nurses also had less choice when their employer required them for special tasks, such as special care or intensive care, where the ability to carry out defined extended roles was a central part of the post and nurses could not therefore refuse.

Another aspect of the original DHSS guidance which does not seem to have survived was the expectation that the doctor was personally delegating that task to a particular nurse, and that the doctor would personally assure the competence of that individual nurse to perform that task. Doctors began to assume that nurses were competent unless they personally protested to the doctor that the task was outside their competence. There might often be no personal contact between the doctor delegating the task and the nurse who performed it. The doctor would give instructions on patient care to the nurse manager who would then allocate the tasks to the ward team. It thus became the responsibility of the ward manager to ensure that tasks were appropriately allocated, and the concept that one task was a medical task (but temporarily delegated to a nurse) and another was basic nursing was lost.

What has survived is the concept of proving competence. When the delegating doctor was required to be personally satisfied that the task was one which the nurse was competent to perform then some form of proof in writing was usual: a certificate of competence or the name listed in a register of competent nurses set up by the employer. Even though the doctor may rarely check an individual nurse's ability to perform a specific task, the nurse might still require this proof of competence, usually in the form of attending a particular training seminar, as an indication of competency.

The Scope of Professional Practice

The publication of *The Scope of Professional Practice* by the UKCC can be seen as a further development of the extended role concept. Its main features can be briefly summarised as follows:

(1)   the term 'extended role' is no longer deemed suitable;

(2)   the emphasis should be on the holistic role of the practitioner not on activities;

(3)   practice must be dynamic and develop with changing needs;

(4)   principles for practice, not certificates for tasks, should form the basis for adjustments to the scope of practice; and

(5)   registration and the Code of Professional Conduct are central to the accountability of the nurse and the Code is the bedrock for judging changes to the scope of professional practice.

The principles on which any development in the scope of practice must develop are as follows:

(1)   the interests of the client/patient must predominate;

(2)   the practitioner must maintain her knowledge, skill and competence;

(3)   the practitioner must also acknowledge the limits of her knowledge, skill and competence;

(4)   the practitioner must not jeopardise standards and must comply with the Code;

(5)   the practitioner must recognise her direct and personal accountability;

(6)   the practitioner must avoid inappropriate delegation.

The implementation of these principles means a radical departure from the traditional role of the nurse and doctor–nurse relationship. The following would be the main effects:

(1)   The traditional demarcation between doctor and nurse would disappear and the main distinctions would reside in their different statutory positions. Certain tasks can only be performed by a registered medical practitioner and these are discussed below.

(2)   There would no longer be a category of functions which the nurse though competent could refuse to perform since she had not the time and they were primarily tasks/activities to be performed by doctors.

(3)   Employers would no longer test competency by looking for certificates.

(4)   The idea of certain tasks being delegated would cease to exist (apart from the registered practitioner to the health care assistant).

There are major legal issues which arise from these changes and they include the following:

(1) What are the legal restrictions which determine which professional can perform a specific activity?

(2) How is competency determined? By the practitioner themself? By the profession? By the employer?

(3) How is liability determined?

(4) How can standards of practice be maintained when the practitioner is under considerable pressure?

(5) How can a practitioner be protected when asserting her incompetence or protesting about falling standards?

(6) What will be the relationship of the nurse practitioner and the junior doctor and other professions?

(7) How will 'in the course of employment' be defined?

(8) If a registered practitioner will be regarded as such even when not employed as such, how can they protect themselves against the pressures of unscrupulous employers?

Legal restrictions

What are the legal restrictions upon the nurse performing specific tasks? Some statutes make it clear that only specific registered persons are entitled to perform specific tasks in the health field. The most important are those which relate to the prescribing, administration, procurement and storage of medicines, where the Medicines Act and the Misuse of Drugs Acts and the statutory instruments regulate the professions which can carry out particular functions.

There are other statutory provisions which place responsibilities on specific professions, such as the notification of infectious diseases, visiting the patient following confinements and the Abortion Act. The Mental Health Act also places clear responsibilities upon the responsible medical officer and on the prescribed nurse.

Recently the power of certain designated nurses to prescribe specified medicinal products has been recognised by statute (namely the Medicinal Products (Nurse Prescribing) Act 1992). The statutory instruments to be published will set out the training requirements for a nurse to be eligible to prescribe and list the drugs which are to be covered by these powers.

There is nothing comparable in our legislation to the Californian state law, quoted in Chapter 10, which prohibits nurse-midwives from using any instrument to assist the birth of the child (with the exception of those to clamp and cut the umbilical cord) or from prescribing or administering before or during birth drugs or medications other than laxatives or disinfectants.

For the most part, however, the statute law does not prescribe who is to perform certain health tasks but leaves it to the statutory bodies which are responsible for registration, education, training and professional conduct, to determine their own roles. These statutory bodies include the United Kingdom Central Council of Nursing, Midwifery and Health Visiting, with the National Boards, the General Medical Council, the General Dental Council and the Council for Professions Supplementary to Medicine. Their rules are based on a concept of the role for that particular profession and the educational requirements are linked to that. If a registered member has acted outside the defined scope of the profession or has acted without the appropriate competence and training, then that member can be summoned to appear before the professional conduct committee and answer to a charge of misconduct.

Unless there is specific statutory legislation which requires a specific professional to carry out specific activities, there is considerable freedom for the development of skills which cross traditional lines of demarcation.

Nurses have been under considerable pressure to take on more and more of the roles which have been traditionally seen as medical. Given below is a list of tasks recognised by one health authority in the early 1980s as being defined as extending the role, and which required clear evidence of additional training before the nurse could be regarded as competent to perform them. They were not seen as being part of the basic training even though many of the older nurses who were trained in the early days of the NHS undertook some of the tasks routinely in earlier posts. 'I used to take bloods, perform ear syringing many years ago yet now the authority says I must go on a training course', was a typical complaint of some.

This provides an interesting contrast with other professions. Doctors, after admission to the Colleges, might be called on to undertake cases which involve techniques, knowledge and skills in which they have never been formally examined. They are expected to study some new area of medicine (often in an extremely short time) and, after observing those who have already developed the necessary skills, undertake new tasks on their own. There are not necessarily any formal checks or further examinations to ensure that an individual is competent. It is expected as part of professional development that the individual will keep up to date and there is no requirement to show a certificate of competence to prove knowledge of the new techniques.

More recently there has been a development for doctors, especially general practitioners, to undertake formal sessions of continuing education where credit points are awarded, and these might eventually become a requirement of continued registration. A particular area of media concern recently (BBC 1993) is keyhole surgery, where there are no requirements by the Royal Colleges that a medical practitioner must have completed a course satisfactorily before undertaking this activity.

It is difficult to keep pace with the numerous activities which nurses became skilled in following registration. Some health authorities have attempted to define the extended role tasks. One health authority produced the following list (Pembrokeshire Health Authority, 1985).

(1) Removal of foreign bodies from eyes
(2) Treatment of warts and verrucae
(3) Patch/prick testing OPD
(4) Spirometry
(5) Mantoux/Heaf test
(6) Skin suturing
(7) Vaccinations
(8) Influenza vaccination for staff
(9) Catheterisation
(10) Reinforcing of plaster of Paris
(11) Gastric lavage/oesophageal tube insertion
(12) Use of monitors and placing of electrodes
(13) Use of microscope
(14) Use of ventilators
(15) Defibrillation
(16) Resuscitation and endotracheal intubation of the new born
(17) Tetanus toxoid
(18) Manual removal of faeces
(19) Intubation
(20) Syringing of ears
(21) Venepuncture
(22) Intravenous administration of drugs
(23) Behaviour therapy
(24) Pessary changing
(25) Trephining of nails
(26) Administration of adrenalin
(27) Administration of cytotoxic drugs
(28) Fitting of breast prosthesis.

Each of these activities was further defined in terms of the nursing areas in which the procedure is undertaken and any recommendations relating to the training or the particular level of nurse who could undertake the task.

Chapter 8 gives a table of tasks generally recognised by ICU practitioners as extending the role, and the responses to a survey described showed that a high proportion of ICU nurses considered that many of these tasks should be standard practice. In Chapter 10 Silverton suggests that it is possible for a midwife in the UK to be the sole carer for a mother from the first point of contact with the maternity services up until 28 days after the birth. The recommendations of the Winterton Committee include the further development of the scope and practice of the midwife (Winterton 1992).

The possibility of demarcation disputes does not however lie just between doctors and nurses or midwives. In Chapter 11 Gary Jones mentions the concern expressed by accident and emergency nurses at the development of the ambulance paramedics in the 1980s. In Chapter 8 Last and Self refer to the confusion amongst ICU nurses over whether role extension would increase or decrease the use of technicians in ICU. Some respondents expressed the fear that some employers might refuse to employ an expensive nurse when a technician could be employed instead.

Understanding competence

If the emphasis moves away from certification of tasks and is placed upon skill, knowledge and competence, these issues arise: How does the nurse know when they are competent? How does the employer determine the competence of an individual employee? How do the profession and the courts determine competence?

Determination of competence by the courts

How do the law and the courts define competence? Where cases of negligence are brought and it is alleged that a nurse is in breach of their duty of care, the courts have used a test that has become known as the Bolam Test to ascertain whether there has been a failure to achieve the required standard of care.[2] The name derives from a case heard in 1957 where the judge stated that the standard of care expected is 'the standard of the ordinary skilled man exercising and professing to have that special skill'. The case was concerned with the alleged negligence of medical staff in administering electro-convulsive therapy without an anaesthetic, relaxant drugs or other forms of restraint apart from a mouth gag. The patient suffered severe physical injuries including the dislocation of both hip joints and fractures of the pelvis on both sides. The judge applied the standard as set out above and the defendants were held not to be negligent. Were the same facts to occur today there would be *prima facie* evidence of negligence because of improvements in the standard of care.

The advantage of the Bolam Test is that it changes as standards of care improve and it is measured against the approved accepted standards of the profession at the time the act of the alleged negligence took place. This means that professionals are not expected to be ahead of the contemporary standards or the ones prevailing at the time the case is heard, which may be many years after the actual time of the incident. Another advantage is that it applies to other professions as well as doctors and therefore the activities performed by a nurse would be judged against the standards that nurses would be expected to follow.

What however of the situation when the nurse is carrying out a task or activity which would normally be carried out by a doctor rather than a nurse? Would the nurse be measured against the standard of a nurse or of a doctor? The Court of Appeal considered the issue of individual liability of a team in the case of *Wilsher* v. *Essex Health Authority*.[3] This case involved the administration of oxygen to a premature baby who suffered from many serious disabilities. Part of the evidence was that a house officer had inserted the catheter to measure oxygen levels into a vein rather than an artery thus recording a lower level of oxygen than would otherwise have been the case. In determining the liability of the team as opposed to individuals the Court of Appeal held that there was no concept of team negligence in law. Each individual professional would be held accountable for their individual actions.

The court held that each individual team member could not be required to observe standards demanded of the unit as a whole. It could not be right, for example, to expose a student nurse to an action for negligence for failure to possess the experience of a consultant. The standard of care required was that of the ordinary skilled person exercising and professing to have that special skill, but that standard was to be determined in the context of the particular posts in the unit rather than according to the general rank or status of the people filling the posts, since the duty ought to be tailored to the acts which the doctor had elected to perform rather than to the doctor themself. It followed that inexperience was no defence to an action for negligence.

In determining the liability of junior or inexperienced staff in comparison with those of greater seniority or experience, one judge stated that an inexperienced doctor who was called to exercise a specialist skill and who made a mistake, nevertheless satisfied the necessary standard of care if the advice and help of a superior was sought when necessary. In the Wilsher case the junior doctor had mistakenly sited the catheter for monitoring oxygen into a vein rather than into an artery. He had asked the senior registrar to check what he had done and the senior registrar failed to notice the error. On these facts and applying the Bolam Test the junior doctor had not been negligent but the senior doctor had.

The advantages of these principles to the patient are clear: any action by the patient if harm has resulted from the actions of a health professional cannot be met with a defence of 'that task/activity was undertaken by a junior doctor or someone with very little experience and that is why you have suffered harm'. The patient is entitled to the standard of care which would be expected of the skilled practitioner exercising and professing to have that special skill. It follows therefore that where activities normally undertaken by doctors are delegated to nursing staff, they would be expected to meet the standards that would be required from a doctor were the doctor to perform the task. The patient is entitled to expect and to have the same approved standard of care whether the task is undertaken by a doctor or by a nurse.

The courts recognise that there might be different practices and policies relating to certain treatments and if one body of approved opinion states that X is normal practice, and another body of approved opinion states that Y is accepted practice, the court will not find against the defendant.

It was not sufficient to establish negligence for the plaintiff to show that there was a body of competent professional opinion that considered the decision was wrong, if there was also a body of equally competent professional opinion that supported the decision as having been reasonable in the circumstances.[4]

From these cases the following principles emerge:

(1)   The courts are not primarily concerned with whether a task/activity is carried out by a nurse or by a doctor (except of course where there is a statutory requirement to that effect). They will be concerned to learn from experts in the field what standards of care the patient should expect to receive and whether there are any acceptable reasons why they were not present in the particular case.
(2)   It would be for those in overall care of the patient to ensure that these standards were met: either through directly undertaking the activity or supervising others.
(3)   Team liability does not exist as a concept in law.
(4)   Standards are variable and will rise as knowledge and experience develops.
(5)   Essentially the professions develop their own standards but these are subject to the scrutiny of the courts.

(6)   Even though the statute places a particular duty as being that of a
       named profession, it might be possible for this to be carried out
       under supervision of that profession by others.[1]

One of the fears which result from the widening of the scope of professional practice of the nurse is the possibility of increased litigation.
One of the interesting results of the research by Last and Self (Chapter 8)
was that 70% of the ICU nurses responding felt that there was a greater
likelihood of their encountering litigation as a result of role extension. A
similar result might be obtained if they had been questioned about the
development of the scope of professional practice. How competence is
determined by both the profession and the individual practitioner is of
great importance in preventing litigation.

Competence and the profession

The UKCC has a statutory duty to maintain standards of professional
practice, and the *Code of Professional Conduct* constitutes strong guidance to registered practitioners. Whilst it does not have the force of law
it would be used as evidence of what constituted good professional
practice in the hearing of any cases of alleged misconduct by a registered
practitioner before the professional conduct committee. The UKCC and
the National Boards define the standards to be achieved through education centres before a practitioner can be registered and thus determine the level of competence required for specific activities.

Should a case of alleged misconduct come before the UKCC where the
competence of the practitioner to perform a specific activity is in
question, the professional conduct committee would seek to ascertain
the extent to which the six principles which form the basis of the
development of professional practice have been followed.

Determining competence is not, however, an easy task, as illu-
strated in Chapters 3, 6 and 11. In Chapter 11 Jones describes a clinical development programme of four levels, and concludes that no one
model of nursing is right for accident and emergency nursing. As Ashworth and Morrison point out in Chapter 3, the determination of competencies may be a superficial exercise. The three broad categories of
activity described in Chapter 6 might still remain the underlying classification of activities for the foreseeable future: activities performed by
nurses in their own right; activities delegated by doctors and which
may be performed without the doctor being present; and activities
delegated by doctors and which may only be performed in their presence.

Competence and the individual practitioner

The nurse will still need to rely heavily upon the professional assessment of competence and in this respect there is a danger that the scope of professional practice might have left the nurse in a vulnerable position.

In the past the nurse has been able to say, 'If I have been on a ENB/ WNB etc. approved course to do A then I am competent. I have my certificate to prove it'. This certificate was therefore the proof to future employers and to the delegating doctor that the nurse could be entrusted with a particular activity/task/role.

In future, with the move away from individual certification for separate tasks, it will not always be easy for the practitioner or for others to determine whether the nurse now has the skill, competence and knowledge to undertake particular functions not included in their initial pre-registration training. Whilst it might be possible to deal competently with an activity as a result of learning from an experienced colleague and be able to cope adequately with 88% of the situations likely to arise, the nurse might have no knowledge or ability to cope with the other 12%.

Obviously there must be considerable supervision by those who are experienced until the practitioner is deemed competent; but has not this always been the case?

The UKCC statement makes it clear that the ultimate responsibility is upon the practitioner to determine their own individual competence and to be prepared to refuse to undertake a task if this confidence is not possessed. This will become increasingly important as certificates and their like cease to be the accepted currency for competence determination. It is interesting to note that the Last and Self survey (Chapter 8) revealed a desire by a high proportion of ICU nurses to retain some form of certification as proof of competence: 87.8% said that they felt that the system of certification was necessary. Some respondents pointed out the need for more guidelines to clarify what is competent.

Competence and the employer

An express or implied term of the contract of employment is that the employee will obey the reasonable orders of the employer. In addition the employee will be expected to undertake their work with reasonable care and skill. If the employee fails to keep these terms of the contract then the employer can take disciplinary measures against the employee and if circumstances justify can terminate the contract of employment by dismissing the employee with or without notice. Competence or the use of reasonable skill would be interpreted by the courts in accordance with the appropriate professional standards.

Some contracts of employment have incorporated the *Code of Professional Conduct* of the UKCC as being a requirement of registered nurse employees. The *Nursing Times* recently undertook a survey to ascertain which NHS authorities, including NHS Trusts, regarded obedience to the Code of Professional Conduct as a term of the contract of employment (Cole 1991). The results showed that a very high proportion did so, particularly amongst the NHS Trusts.

However, there is a danger that disputes could arise between employer and employee over the definition of competence, with pressure being placed upon the employee to accept insufficient training and experience before carrying out additional activities. For example, a midwife might be expected to carry out obstetric ultrasound after minimal experience. This is a task for which, as Silverton points out in Chapter 10, a radiographer requires 18 months of post-qualification diploma courses.

Similarly, Gary Jones points out in Chapter 11 that a study by the Royal Colleges of Radiologists, Radiographers and Nursing and the British Medical Association has shown that it is safe for accident and emergency nurses to request x-ray examinations prior to the patients seeing the doctor and that this reduces the overall time the patient spends in the department. There is a danger that the unscrupulous employer will not make sufficient investment in the necessary training.

As a result of the internal market and the creation of NHS Trusts we are now seeing the production of protocols by Trusts or GP Fundholders on the clinical responsibilities of nurses. These include many duties formerly carried out by junior doctors. However, if they do not conflict with any statutory provision and if the nurse is given the necessary training and support from the doctor then there is nothing illegal about them.

As a result the nurse practitioner in 10 years time might be a specialist very different from that of today. A nurse might, for example, have a training in skills normally used by a physiotherapist, some normally used by a junior houseman on a surgical ward and possibly also be able to carry out diagnostic tests such as ECGs and others.

Unfortunately not all employers are scrupulous in ensuring that their employees have the relevant training, knowledge and competence before they are asked to undertake particular tasks. Examples can be found particularly amongst practice nurses who have been asked to perform tasks without adequate training. Nurses who are employed by general practitioners are extremely vulnerable since a refusal to undertake a particular activity could cost them their jobs.

How is liability determined?

By the courts?

Competence, the standard of care and the laws of negligence go hand in hand in determining civil liability. If a practitioner has failed to follow the approved standard of care which would reasonably be expected of a professional and harm has been foreseeably caused as a result then there would be liability.

If a nurse carries out any activities negligently: (a) the nurse could be personally liable; (b) the employer would be vicariously liable; (c) if the nurse failed to have adequate training for the task being undertaken, the manager or the person who asked them to carry out the task might be liable as well.

By the profession?

The Professional Conduct Committee of the UKCC has the task of first determining if the conduct of which the nurse has been found guilty is properly defined as misconduct and secondly if so what should be the outcome.

Increasingly the UKCC has not looked at events in isolation, but where the practitioner has not been supported by management officers then they have come in for disciplinary action as well. Central to the determination of misconduct would be whether the practitioner was acting outside their field of competence. The practitioner can therefore look to the UKCC for help if undue pressure is brought to bear upon them.

Maintaining standards

The practitioner, knowing their own field of competence and being aware of the professional standards expected, has a major role to play in the determination and the maintenance of standards in the new scenario of the purchaser/provider divide.

In one respect the internal market makes the task easier because at the heart of the NHS agreements between providers and purchasers there must be terms covering both the quantity and the quality of services to be provided, and the practitioner has a major role to play in the setting and the monitoring of these.

The Secretary of State has recently announced that there will be a channel of communication for those within the NHS who are potential whistleblowers, that is, those who believe that hazardous practices are taking place and there is no obvious action or concern by management. They will be able to raise these issues without fear of victimisation. The NHS Management Executive has produced guidance for staff on relations with the public and the media (DoH 1993). This emphasises in bold print that 'in no circumstances are employees who express their views about health service issues in accordance with this guidance to be penalised in any way for doing so'. Still, the guidance might be regarded as unduly restrictive by some staff. It might not be sufficient to protect staff who complain of lowering standards, who might remain vulnerable to the loss of jobs and therefore require the protection of such bodies as the UKCC.

How can the practitioner be protected when asserting that they are incompetent to perform specific roles or when protesting about declining standards? This is a real issue facing many practitioners. The Secretary of State at a conference in July 1992 undertook to set up an internal complaints mechanism, so that staff who are concerned about the standards of care or other ways in which their professional code of conduct cannot be kept, would be able to make known their concerns to the senior levels of management and not be scapegoated. It would appear that the guidance mentioned above (DoH 1993) is intended to cover this.

Staff are vulnerable. Those who have recently been employed by NHS Trusts may not have the two years minimum service necessary to bring an action for unfair dismissal. Raising justified grievances may therefore put their posts in jeopardy. They cannot necessarily look to colleagues for support. Strike action or any industrial work to rule is ethically not acceptable to many practitioners and indeed can be said to be contrary to the Code of Professional Conduct. There are no signs that the UKCC is able or prepared to take public action for those practitioners who find themselves in a Catch 22 dilemma. This is a serious situation and one which should be considered by the Government and the statutory bodies in order to ensure that standards are maintained.

Rowley points out in Chapter 9, in relation to practice nurses, that as the localised extended role certificates are abolished following the release of the UKCC's *The Scope of Professional Practice*, saying 'No' to GPs who ask them to carry out tasks for which they have not been trained could become more difficult than ever. Silverton (Chapter 10) is concerned that the reduction in the hours of junior doctors has been followed by an examination of who should do what in the field of hospital-based health care. This has coincided with a reduction in hospital-based antenatal clinics and the realisation that some 'medical tasks' were actually prompted by midwives.

Nurse and junior doctor

What will be the relationship of the nurse practitioner and junior doctor? This is an interesting area since it is clear from the clinical protocols being developed that nurse practitioners are being used to undertake work often carried out by junior doctors as part of their training. There has often been an anomaly between the function of a nurse in a medical teaching hospital and one in a non-teaching hospital.

It is likely that as part of the developments within the NHS specific hospitals will receive extra funds for taking part in the training of doctors. Similarly there may be contracts for hospitals to provide clinical placements for nurses on the Project 2000 training courses. Where such contracts exist for these training purposes then the staff may have different roles in relation to the trainees.

There is discussion taking place over whether the present post of hospital consultant should be abolished and two grades created in its place: specialist and senior specialist (NAHAT 1992). Whatever the outcome, there are likely to be some radical changes in relation to the training of junior doctors and the related position of the clinical nurse practitioner.

As the role of the clinical nurse practitioner develops there will need to be clarification of the work of the nurse *vis à vis* the junior doctor, and the nurse will need support and protection.

Course of employment

How will 'in the course of employment' be defined? It will still be the responsibility of the employer to define the title and job content of his employees' contracts of employment. There may well be greater flexibility over this than in the past unless the individual professional groups commence demarcation disputes.

Statutory support however would be required to ensure that, for example, tasks which were normally performed by a registered physiotherapist continued to be performed only by a registered member of that profession.

Course of employment is simply what the employer agrees to the employee undertaking, providing it is not contrary to the law. The employer cannot turn a blind eye to what the employee is actually doing and cannot, in defence of an action for the vicarious liability of the employer for the employee's negligence, argue that the work was done outside their wishes. They would still be liable.

Even where the employer has expressly prohibited an employee from carrying out a particular task or instructed that it should be performed in a particular way, and the employee disobeys these instructions, the employer may still be vicariously liable for any harm caused by the employee whilst working on the employers behalf.[5]

If a registered practitioner is not employed as such, but an unscrupulous employer wishes to take advantage of skills for which she is not employed, how can she be protected? This is a real possibility since the UKCC document emphasises that even though not employed as such, a registered practitioner must still follow the accepted standards of the profession and the Code of Professional Conduct. It is possible therefore for a practitioner to be employed in a residential home as a care assistant or manager and the employer to make use of their skills as a registered nurse even though the employer is not paying for those skills.

In this situation it is for the practitioners to defend themselves through their own organisations to prevent exploitation. What is clear is that the UKCC would not allow any falling off of standards.

Conclusion

A new era has arrived in health care. Traditional demarcation lines are disappearing. The internal market has established new relationships and thinking. The UKCC document, *The Scope of Professional Practice*, has shown the lead in enabling practitioners to adapt to these changes on the basis of clearly defined principles.

If there is abuse of the flexibility that is at present permitted by the law then it may be that new statutory rules will be required to specify who can do what. Until that time the existing laws and the professional conduct procedures of the professions will have to ensure that the public is protected and the practitioners have the support they require to maintain and raise standards of care.

Any experimentation in the role of the nurse practitioner should be accompanied by clear guidelines on procedures and training and an understanding that the performance of individual activities must be underpinned by a substantial foundation of education and understanding. The practitioners' role must be seen in the context of this foundation and not as a collection of *ad hoc* tasks.

Notes

1 Royal College of Nurses *v.* The Department of Health and Social Security [1981] 1 All ER 545.

2　Bolam *v.* Friern HMC [1957] 2 All ER 118.
3　Wilsher *v.* Essex Area Health Authority CA [1986] 3 All ER 801.
4　Maynard *v.* West Midlands Regional Health Authority [1984] 1 WLR 634.
5　Century Insurance Co. Ltd *v.* Northern Ireland Road Transport Board [1942] 1 All ER 491.

References

BBC (1993) *Panorama* programme, 23 June. British Broadcasting Corporation, London.

Cole A. (1991) Nursing Times Survey. *Nursing Times* **87** (27), 26.

Department of Health and Social Security (1977) Circular HC(77)22. DHSS, London.

Department of Health and Social Security (1989) Letters PL/CMO(89)7 and PL/CNO(89)10. DHSS, London (see Appendix V in this volume).

Department of Health (1993) *Guidance for Staff on Relations with the Public and the Media*, EL(93)51. NHS Management Executive, London.

NAHAT (1992) Proposals, September 1992. National Association of Health Authorities and Trusts, London.

Pembrokeshire H. A. (1985) Circular list of extended role tasks in nursing, December.

Winterton (1992) *The Report of the House of Commons Select Committee on Maternity Services*, February 1992, London.

Chapter 5
Nurse Prescribing

Introduction

The enhancement of nursing practice and the fulfilment of nursing potential demands a continuous review of professional activities in order that the changing health needs of the population may be effectively met. Nurses must constantly be prepared to move into areas of practice which will maximise their healing role, and undertake research and evaluation to achieve the best possible health for patients and clients. Enabling nurses to prescribe is a significant development among the many changes currently occurring within the profession.

The discrete activity of prescribing must be set within the context of professional nursing, which is 'the provision of care as a dynamic process which has the patient's health as the objective [and] is reflected in such aspects as individual self care ability, self esteem and self determination' (McMahon 1991). Nurse prescribing allows patients to be effectively and speedily treated in health centres and the home, the workplace and at school by practitioners. Prescribing may be included within the range of instrumental skills described by Wright (1991) which, when combined with the 'high touch' expressive skills which are the essence of nursing, provide 'a healing role which serves the patient'.

The legislative process, which was completed with the passage of the Medicinal Products: Prescription by Nurses, etc. Bill (1992), empowers suitably qualified nurses, midwives and health visitors to undertake the independent activity of prescribing from the Nurses' Formulary. Together with named specialist nurses they will also be able to alter the timing and dosage of medications prescribed by medical practitioners within clearly defined protocols. This is particularly important when, for example, people with complex or unstable conditions, such as those who are terminally ill, are being cared for at home.

General requirements

To prescribe effectively nurses will need:

(1) an increased awareness of professional accountability;
(2) a full understanding of the process of assessment and diagnosis that results in the act of prescribing;
(3) a knowledge of therapeutics and practical prescribing (Andrews 1992).

Nurses who assume teaching as well as practice responsibilities will need to take account of their patient's past health history, and current and anticipated health status. Thorough knowledge of the item to be prescribed, its action, side effects, dosage and frequency of use in a variety of circumstances will also be essential. Nurses will be required to develop and maintain their current knowledge base in pharmacology, physiology, disease and illness processes, therapeutics and practical prescribing (Fig. 5.1). They will need to apply this at the same time as taking account of the socio-economic and psychological needs of patients and their legal and administrative responsibilities as prescribers.

- Past health history
- Current and anticipated health status
- Knowledge of item to be prescribed:
  action, side-effects, dosage and frequency of use
- Knowledge of underlying illness
- Details related to practical prescribing
- Legal and administrative responsibilities
- Professional responsibilities

Fig. 5.1 Factors to be taken into account by nurses who prescribe.

It is clear that nurses who will be empowered to prescribe must have undertaken the necessary education and training and have a record to that effect on the Register of the United Kingdom Central Council for Nursing, Midwifery and Health Visiting (UKCC). This is essential in order that the public is served by properly prepared practitioners and in the interest of public safety.

A humanistic approach

Nurse prescribing is an acknowledgement and endorsement of the current contribution of nurses to patient care, and a recognition of the need to supply items necessary for effective nursing treatment (Andrews 1992). While it will clearly be necessary for medical practitioners, nurse prescribers and pharmacists to collaborate closely in the prescribing process to ensure safe practice, the current costly, demeaning and unnecessarily delaying practice of awaiting medical confirmation of the independent nursing decision will be eliminated.

A cost benefit analysis (DoH 1991) has suggested an initial investment of between £13m and £17m is required to ensure the educational preparation of the nurses involved, but this will be outweighed by the particular advantages prescribing will bring to patients and clients. Some of these were outlined in the Report of the Advisory Group on Nurse Prescribing (The Crown Report) and include:

(1) a service which is more appropriate and responsive to patients' needs;
(2) better, faster more cost effective treatment of minor, but potentially serious and therefore costly conditions;
(3) more appropriate use of nurses' extensive professional skills;
(4) less wastage with more appropriate treatment; and
(5) less travelling and consequent saving of time and other attached costs (DoH 1989c).

Further advantage may be gained by the fundamentally different orientation of nurses, who view the individual as a whole, with emphasis on that individual's own perspective. Nurses focus on health promotion and facilitate self-care with their patients and clients. The primary role of nursing is to enable independence and interdependence, and the discrete activity of prescribing must be seen in this context.

When prescribing, supplying or altering the timing or dosage of an item nurses will have the opportunity to actively engage in health teaching with the potential benefit of enabling people to become self-caring. Nurses will ask whether any prescription is required at all. As Smith and Ross (1992), McMahon (1991) and others have pointed out, they are already skilled in many other therapeutic options and the decision to prescribe additional drugs or other items should always take account of the risks and benefits of therapy.

Many items included in the suggested Nurses' Formulary are readily available 'over the counter' but, as Smith and Ross (1992) suggest, patients will take the safety of such products for granted when they are prescribed by a nurse, as is currently the case when they are prescribed by the doctor. Members of the public expect infinitely more knowledge and expertise from a nurse who prescribes than when choosing a product for themselves.

When combined with the potential for health teaching, the activity of nurse prescribing takes on extra significance. In the area where nurses have shown most interest in prescribing – simple analgesics, topical applications, wound dressings, incontinence products, bandages and tapes – there is the greatest opportunity to combine this intervention with health education. The prescribed product is introduced on the understanding that the end goal is self-care or carer action with the item readily available through a community pharmaceutical outlet.

Further responsibilities will be expected of nurses who assume the authority of teaching others about products which, if used incorrectly, could do more harm than good. In anticipation of such advanced nursing responsibilities the UKCC (1992a) has made adjustments to the Code of Conduct stating:

> 'As a registered nurse, midwife or health visitor, you are personally accountable for your practice and, in the exercise of your professional accountability, must: work in an open and co-operative manner with patients, clients and their families, foster their independence and recognise and respect their involvement in the planning and delivery of care.'

The Council has issued additional guidance on role enhancement in its publication on *The Scope of Professional Practice* (UKCC 1992b). Principles for adjusting the dimensions of practice have been laid down which should, in future, form the basis upon which each practitioner may base her or his decision when considering any extension or expansion of professional responsibility. These principles are set out in Appendix I.

The Crown Report

The health needs of defined populations are the starting point for all matters relating to health care provision. The need to fulfil the prescribing requirement of people living in the community more efficiently was the starting point for the Advisory Group which, under the direction of Dr June Crown, set about tackling the complex remit given to them. The Secretary of State had asked for recommendations on:

(1) the circumstances in which nurses might prescribe, order or supply drugs, dressings, appliances and chemical reagents;
(2) the categories of items which might properly be ordered or supplied by nurses, and the arrangements needed to sustain such activities;
(3) the methods by which drugs, etc. might be prescribed;
(4) the circumstances in which a nurse may properly vary the timing and dosage of drugs prescribed;

(5)   to advise on the implications of the recommendations for training; and

(6)   to consider resource implications (DoH 1989c).

The first formal acknowledgement that an investigation into the extent and nature of nurse prescribing in the United Kingdom was required may be found in the Cumberlege Report (1986). This seminal work recognised that nurses undertaking their central role of providing therapeutic care for people in the community were unable to prescribe the items they needed for effective care. However highly skilled these nurses were they were required to ask a registered medical practitioner to write out a prescription. The findings of Cumberlege accord with similar evidence from the USA where a recently published survey suggests that 'the health care system desperately needs the competent, cost effective primary care provided by nursing practitioners', but that 'frustrating barriers', including 'limits on practice and prescriptive authority', prevent large numbers of advanced practice nurses from working efficiently and discourage them from staying in the field (Pearson 1992).

In the UK and the USA studies have demonstrated nurse competence in the prescribing activity, and the Crown Report indicated that prevailing British constraints resulted in community nurses being involved in excessive travel, time lapse and therefore unnecessary cost.

The nurse time taken to process prescription items such as dressings, antiseptics and catheters, that in previous administrative systems had been readily available in the community and continued to be immediately accessible to nurses in hospital, could be saved if nurses were able to prescribe items themselves. To ask general practitioners to prescribe in such circumstances was seen by the Advisory Group as leading to lack of clarity about professional responsibilities and as demeaning to both nurses and doctors (DoH 1989c).

The Group specifically set out to address the Cumberlege recommendations to make better use of community nursing skills:

'The DHSS should agree a limited list of items and simple agents which may be prescribed by nurses as part of a nursing care programme and issue guidelines to enable nurses to control drug dosage in well-defined circumstances' (Cumberlege 1986, p.33).

The Cumberlege Report was immediately followed by another report which also recommended that nurses should prescribe from a limited formulary.

Throughout their work the Nurse Prescribing Advisory Group took as their guiding principle 'the consideration of what is best for patient care both in terms of clinical effectiveness and convenience for their patients and their carers' (DoH 1989c, 1. 11). The Group went on to make 27 recommendations which were addressed to the Department of Health, the UKCC, Health Authorities and the professions (Appendix II in this volume). These recommendations relate to six core areas of:

- practice
- education
- administration
- legal issues
- communication
- public safeguards.

All these areas are related and, since publication of the nurse prescribing report, have been variously addressed by the bodies which are currently undertaking preparatory work to enable the commencement of nurse prescribing.

Definition and limitations

The definition of the word 'prescribe' given in the *Collins English Dictionary and Thesaurus* (1987) is: 'to lay down as a rule or directive; to recommend or order the use of'. It is clear that nurses already do these in relation to the independent and collaborative activity of nursing practice. Nurses make nursing diagnoses and decisions continuously and advise patients, clients and carers accordingly. The Crown Report relates specifically to the expansion of those activities into areas relating to the prescription of drugs, dressings, applications, and chemical reagents which are used as part of care.

The Report recommended that only those nurses with a UKCC recognised qualification in district nursing or health visiting might be authorised to undertake the independent activity of prescribing. The Report also proposed that stoma care nurses, continence advisors, diabetic liaison nurses, terminal care (palliative care) nurses, community psychiatric nurses and community mental handicap nurses might not prescribe directly. Such nurses could, in certain circumstances, alter the timing and dosage of drugs and supply items within predetermined protocols.

Since publication of the report those groups of nurses who, together with district nurses and health visitors, form part of the primary health care nursing service but have not been accorded prescribing rights, have questioned the wisdom of singling out those with district nurse and health visitor qualifications to undertake this activity. It seems likely that with acceptance and progression of the principles outlined by the UKCC in *The Code of Professional Conduct* (1992a); *The Scope of Professional Practice* (1992b); and *The Community Education and Practice Report* (UKCC 1991); combined with the broad remit of the Medicinal Products: Prescription by Nurses, etc. Bill (1992), the range and number of nurses empowered to prescribe will increase.

Preparing nurses for prescribing

In deciding who might prescribe and in what circumstances, it is necessary to acknowledge that pharmaceutical prescribing is a complex activity. Rawlings (1991) explored the necessity for nurses having a comprehensive knowledge of drugs, dressings and wound management treatments before commencing with prescribing. Pearson (1992) found that in the USA nurses with prescribing powers required extensive preparatory education. Statutory regulations vary from State to State but, for example, in California nurses must register as prescribers upon completion of a pharmacology course and a 6-month preceptorship with a physician. In Connecticut 'nurse practitioners, clinical specialists, nurse midwives and nurse anaesthetists may apply for prescriptive practice privileges', following statutory national certification, completion of 30 hours pharmacology and a masters degree, (regulations to come into force in 1994). In other States (e.g. Idaho, Kentucky and New Jersey) nurses may undertake derivative or dependent prescribing within protocols determined by medical practitioners (Pearson 1992).

Whether in the USA or the UK, or indeed anywhere else in the world, nurses must be fully aware of and prepared for the implications of nurse prescribing in terms of autonomy, responsibility, and authority, all based on individual assessment and care requirements. Nurses embarking upon prescribing must assume personal responsibility for ensuring they have fulfilled their professional obligations set out in the Code of Conduct (UKCC 1992a) and have received appropriate education, are assessed as competent, and have the outcome of that assessment recorded in such a way that it is readily available to *bona fide* enquirers such as pharmacists.

The Nurses, Midwives and Health Visitors Act (1992) envisaged that the UKCC, as the competent authority, would utilise its Register to fulfil the recording requirement, and it is reasonable to assume that the final outcomes of the Post-Registration Education and Practice Project will include appropriate mechanisms to ensure public safety in relation to nurse prescribing. The Crown Report determined that at the time of preparation (1987–88) health visitors and district nurses were the only nurses, in addition to midwives who already had prescribing authority, immediately likely to meet the requirements. The Report recommended evaluation and extension to other groups over time, and it was hoped that extension might be secured in time for the commencement of prescribing in 1993.

Legislation

In recommending that nurses assume responsibility for prescribing, the Crown Report identified the need for an amendment to Section 41 of the NHS Act (1977) and a further need to alter legislation providing exemption to part of the Medicines Act 1968. The Report also highlighted the necessity for establishing systems to take account of the legal liability consequent on nurses prescribing, such as indemnity insurance, and the local determination of prescribing protocols.

Since the Crown Report was published the new Government White Papers, *Working for Patients* (DoH 1989a) and *Caring for People* (DoH 1989b), have led to the NHS Act 1992 and the passage of the Medicinal Products: Prescription by Nurses, etc., Bill (1992). The main purpose of the Bill is to enable retail pharmacists to dispense medicinal products listed in the Nurses Formulary (awaited) which arose from 'prescriptions issued by certain categories of nurses, midwives and health visitors'.

Clause 1 of the Bill specifies that registered nurses, midwives and health visitors are 'appropriate practitioners' for the purpose of prescribing 'prescription only medicines' under Section 58 of the Medicines Act 1968. It gives powers to Ministers to limit the categories of nurses, midwives and health visitors who may prescribe by reference to qualifications and training. Clause 1 also gives power to Ministers to prohibit an 'appropriate practitioner' who is a nurse, midwife or health visitor from delegating the administration parenterally of prescription only medicinal products to others.

Clauses 2, 3 and 4 of the Bill amend Section 41 of the NHS Act 1977 and a similar clause of the NHS (Scotland) Act 1978 and provide for an order in Council for Northern Ireland so that the Family Health Service Authorities and similar bodies arrange for the provision of pharmaceutical services in the same way that they are already provided for general practitioners and dentists.

The legislation is necessary to ensure that only properly educated nurses may undertake the responsibility for prescribing products which

are potentially harmful if used indiscriminately by those without sufficient knowledge and competence.

Nurses who engage in the activity of prescribing medicinal products
will need to assume legal responsibilities. (Wider legal aspects of role
expansion are discussed in Chapter 4.) These include an understanding
of the duty of care every nurse has towards patients and clients and the
consequences inherent upon inappropriate or negligent prescribing
actions. The matter of vicarious liability will need to be explored, particularly where a GP and a nurse are sharing responsibility for providing
prescriptions for patients.

One of the real benefits to ensue from this will be the essential
requirement for shared records to minimise the possibility of confusion
about individuals and shared responsibilities where prescribing is concerned. Because nurses will increasingly assume responsibility for their
own actions it will also be essential for individual nurses and professional bodies to explore and develop the extent of professional indemnity insurance.

The process of nurse prescribing

The activity of reaching a decision about the use of a product and the
practical details that surround the ordering, dispensing and administration of these products is secondary to the primary decision-making
process involving diagnosis. Diagnosis is the reaching of a conclusion
about the nature and cause of a condition from a collection of 'symptoms' or presenting occurrences.

As with the activity of prescribing, diagnosis is more usually associated with the practice of medicine, although the differential decision-
making between a range of possibilities as to the cause of a presenting
problem is a fundamental human activity which only requires the
expertise of professional intervention in the most serious or unusual
situations. For example, all mothers make differential diagnosis as to the
cause of their children's coughs, sneezes, rashes, aches and pains, and in
adulthood the same process is undertaken as a self-care activity. Diagnosis may therefore be undertaken by nurses when the decision-making
involves the distinctive practice of nursing in the same way that medical
practitioners use the process when dealing with serious disease.

Factors which must be taken into account when assessing any individual health state with a view to reaching a diagnosis and prescribing
treatment are set out in Fig. 5.2.

Nurses will learn to make differential diagnoses between similar
conditions reaching an appropriate diagnosis using symptoms, observed

- Age and stage of life and the individual
- Causes, duration and frequency of the symptoms
- Functional impairment resulting from the condition
- Impairment of life quality resulting from the condition
- Manifestations of disturbance:
  physical, behavioural and emotional
- History and predisposing factors
- Family history/patterns

Fig. 5.2   Factors to be taken into account when assessing any individual health state.

signs, technological and biochemical testing as a guide. Many district nurses are already highly proficient in the management of, for example, leg ulcers using Doppler technology to assist with diagnosis, following which appropriate management regimes may then be implemented.

Once a diagnosis has been reached a further, secondary judgement must be made about which product, if any, might be useful as an adjunct to treatment. Before proceeding to assume responsibility for ordering a substance which could potentially be harmful to the patient the nurse must have sufficiently comprehensive pharmacological knowledge. No nurse, doctor or other health professional should prescribe a product without having a full understanding of the product's attributes (see Fig. 5.3).

Every nurse will need to consider their personal responsibilities under the UKCC Code of Conduct with regard to acquiring sufficiently detailed knowledge. This form of personal professional development will be ongoing throughout a career lifetime to take account of the frequent emergence of new products on the market.

Nurses will also need to become proficient at discerning the best

- Composition
- Physical properties
- Absorption
- Fate in the body
- Method of excretion
- Effects on cells and systems (including social systems)
- Acute and chronic toxicity
- Uses and advantages
- Effectiveness
- Preparation and dosage
- Ease of procurement
- Cost

Fig. 5.3   Factors which must be taken into account before prescribing a product.

products available from the wealth of marketing literature which is likely to be produced by pharmaceutical companies. Nurses will need to share this experience with GPs. Team working will facilitate ethical decision-making in the best interests of patients and clients.

Conclusions

Good communication between various professional groups was seen as a crucial issue by the Working Group led by Dr June Crown who presented the original Nurse Prescribing Report. It is especially important in clinical audit processes to test and demonstrate the effectiveness of nurse prescribing. There will need to be good communications between doctors, nurses and pharmacists with highly efficient shared systems of records if nurse prescribing is to work. Each professional group will need to be particularly vigilant to ensure multiple and possibly conflicting prescriptions are not issued. In the best circumstances, shared audit and shared statements of good practice will result.

New possibilities are created for nurses and pharmacists to work more closely together. One example is the Nurse Practitioner Project currently under way in the South East Thames Region where a nurse is holding consulting sessions in a community pharmacist's retail outlet (South East Thames Regional Health Authority 1992). Further development in the area of patient-held records may reduce delay when several people are prescribing for one patient.

It is envisaged that nurse prescribing will result in better, faster, more cost-effective treatment of minor, but potentially serious (and therefore costly) conditions. Nurse prescribing should promote the development of a service which is more responsive to patients' needs and make better use of expensive professional skills, with less wastage and more appropriate treatment.

Careful evaluation of the first projects will be required to see if these expectations are met. It may then be that the right to prescribe becomes a routine function for all registered nurses.

References

Andrews S. (1992) Prescription for Success. *Health Direct* March, 12.
Cumberlege Report (1986) *Neighbour Nursing – A Focus for Care.* DHSS, London.
Department of Health/Touche Ross (1991) *Nurse Prescribing: Final Report A Cost Benefit Study.* DoH, London.

Department of Health (1989a) *Working for Patients* (CM555). DoH, London.

Department of Health (1989b) *Caring for People* (CM849). DoH, London.

Department of Health (1989c) *Report of the Advisory Group on Nurse Prescribing: The Crown Report.* DoH, London.

McMahon R. (1991) Therapeutic nursing, theory, issues and practice. In *Nursing as Therapy* (eds R. McMahon & A. Pearson). Chapman Hall, London.

Pearson L. J. (1992) 1991–92 update: how each state stands on legislative issues affecting advanced nursing practice. *Nurse Practitioner: The American Journal of Primary Health Care* **17** (1), 156–67.

Rawlings M. (1991) Nurse prescribing – a pharmacist's view. Paper presented at Nursing Times Conference, Manchester, June 1991.

Smith F. & Ross F. (1992) Prescribing for pain. *Community Outlook* **10**, 4–5.

South East Thames Regional Health Authority (1992) *People for Health, Health for People: Nurse Practitioner Projects 1992–1994.* SETHRA, East Sussex.

United Kingdom Central Council for Nursing, Midwifery and Health Visiting (1991) *Report on the Proposals for the Future of Community Education and Practice.* UKCC, London.

United Kingdom Central Council for Nursing, Midwifery and Health Visiting (1992a) *Code of Professional Conduct for the Nurse, Midwife and Health Visitor.* UKCC, London.

United Kingdom Central Council for Nursing, Midwifery and Health Visiting (1992b) *The Scope of Professional Practice for the Nurse, Midwife and Health Visitor.* UKCC, London.

Wright S. (1991) Facilitating therapeutic nursing and independent practice. In *Nursing as Therapy* (eds R. McMahon & A. Pearson). Chapman Hall, London.

Chapter 6
European Aspects of the Nursing Role

Introduction

The purpose of this chapter is to explore the role of the nurse in the European context with specific reference to the concepts of role expansion and extension.

Europe is defined as that geographical area covered by the World Health Organization's European Regional Office. In view of the major political upheavals in the so-called Eastern Bloc, no attempt will be made to list the existing and emerging states within the Region.

Rogers (1991) has identified the diversity in the make-up of the health care work forces throughout Europe. Nursing forms the largest single group of health care workers in most countries and yet there are major differences in the definitions of the role, education and status of the nurse within and between the European States. It is only within the European Community (EC) that there has been an attempt to standardise the education of nurses (Quinn 1982).

The Single European Act 1986 will create a new marketplace for nursing services. The removal of national frontiers regulating the flow of capital, goods, services and people within the EC could result in a redistribution of nurses. This raises issues concerning the supply of and demand for nurses, their education, and terms and conditions of service. Furthermore, it necessitates a common agreement on the best use of nursing skills to meet the population's changing demands for health care (Paillet-Kelson 1992).

Attempts to compare the demands for and supplies of nurses and the profiles of the nursing services in each European country are beset with problems. The databases held in each country are compiled in different ways and utilise widely differing means of collecting, collating, analysing and storing the data. All that we may assume about nursing practice throughout Europe is that nurses form an integral and substantial part of the health care workforce in each State, albeit in different proportions in each country (WHO 1985; Abel-Smith 1985; OECD 1990).

To counter-balance this confusion, the WHO's document 'Health for all by the Year 2000' (WHO 1978; Asval *et al.* 1986) provides the first comprehensive and concrete international health policy framework for the future. The 38 targets developed by the 33 Member States of the WHO European Region in 1985 provide both policy and strategic intent for the development of nursing services and practice in Europe (WHO 1989). Thus there is for the first time a strategic health care plan and goals for the Region's nursing services, which will unify and strengthen the provision of nursing care in and between the member states. Furthermore, it provides a framework for future collaborative studies in nursing education, practice, management and research (WHO 1988).

The adoption of the WHO targets as the focus for the nursing services in member states will continue to demand a re-negotiation of the role boundaries between nurses and their co-workers in health care organisations, between nurses and informal care givers, and the definition of the support worker. This in turn implies that both role expansion and extension will continue to be a part of the daily practice of the nurse and will raise issues in regard to the direction the profession should take in the future (Caspane *et al.* 1990).

A review of the literature

Access to accurate accounts of what nurses do in their respective jobs in each country is extremely limited. This may reflect the fact that not all nurses record accounts of their practice or have access to publishers, or that if they do publish accounts of their practice it is in the language of their country of origin. The literature reviewed here, therefore, is limited to that published in the English language and in the international nursing journals.

Those articles to which we do have access confine themselves to broad descriptions of the developments of nursing as a profession, the education of the nurse, and to a certain extent the ideal role of the nurse in a specific context. Examples of such literature include: Fagermoen's (1984) account of the nurse education system in Norway; Uyer (1984) and Kum (1972) on the history of nursing in Turkey; Milena's (1972) review of the origins of nursing in Slovenia (formerly part of Yugoslavia); and Diepeveen-Speekenbrink's report (1990) of the innovations in collaborative nursing education between the Netherlands and the United Kingdom.

This broad approach does permit us insights into the roots and development of each nursing service in different countries. Outwardly the diversity of nursing services suggests that there may be little shared by those employed in these services, but the descriptions do reveal common threads running through the structure, function and education of the nurse in Europe.

The origins of modern nursing in the UK are generally agreed to be found in the Nightingale reforms of the mid-nineteenth century (Abel-Smith 1960). Miss Nightingale's work in the Crimea and her visit to Kaiserworth in Germany are well recorded. One could easily gain the impression that Nightingale invented nursing and that she alone influenced its adoption in other countries. However, the review of the literature clearly shows that others visited Kaiserworth, were influenced by the work being carried out there and went back to their own countries to found what are now modern nursing services.

Fagermoen (1984) records just such a visit by the founder of modern nursing in Norway and the creation of a vocational training programme identical to the Nightingale model. Later developments in the Norwegian services may have been influenced by the employment of a Matron trained at the Royal Infirmary in Edinburgh in 1908. Thus, the Nightingale model reinforced that of the Norwegian founder but the primary source of influence came from Kaiserworth in Germany.

The influence of German nursing models is also recorded by Uyer (1984) and Kum (1972) in their separate accounts of the development of the Turkish nursing service. Each of these writers also acknowledges the influence of Nightingale on a Turkish doctor during his visit to London. It is noteworthy that whilst Nightingale received much acclaim for her work in Scutari (Istanbul), she does not appear to have had any direct impact on the local community during her stay in Turkey. Kum (1972), however, draws our attention to the rich historical heritage of the Turkish health service and traces its origins back to Cairo in the 9th Century. Kum also acknowledges the work of the Red Crescent which, like the Red Cross, has done so much to assist the development of nursing services. Badouaille (1972) provides us with accounts of how the Red Cross played an important role in providing postgraduate education for nurses in France as late as 1971.

Milena (1972) in her account of the development of nursing in Slovenia also identifies the influence of the church and the nursing services provided by religious orders in the Austro-Hungarian Empire of the 1780s. The first nursing clinics for mothers and children developed in Slovenia in the early part of this century and trained nurses were in evidence in 1924.

Iceland is perhaps one of the youngest of European nations. The history and culture of its people are clearly linked to that of Norway. It is therefore not surprising that O'Leary (1972) identifies the influence of the Nordic countries on the nursing services in Iceland since their inception in 1919.

From these historical accounts of the development of modern nursing we can conclude that these services: arose from a tradition grounded in religious beliefs (Christian and Islamic); arose in response to a perceived social need; were organised by strong willed and determined individuals; were influenced by the conflicts of the First and Second World Wars; were seen as mainly an occupation for women and therefore closely linked to the changing social status of women in each country; and were heavily controlled through the political economy of health and the medical profession in each country. All of these nursing services originated in hospital-based services and vocational education programmes, and all have spread out beyond the hospital walls to include community-based services. Furthermore, changes in the labour markets and policies on education, health and social welfare are channelling nursing education into the higher education sector throughout Europe.

In the United Kingdom, the Netherlands, Sweden, Turkey, Germany and Finland, departments of nursing are being established in the higher education sector (Olsson & Gulberg 1988; Grauhan 1970; Katajamaki 1970; Deipenveen-Speekenbrink 1990). This move into higher education reflects the demands for a 'knowledgeable doer' who can meet the public's changing demands for health care in the hospital and community setting and provide effective, efficient services to different populations.

From a professional perspective, nurses in the higher education sector throughout Europe are engaging in research activities to establish a clear and well-defined professional role together with recognition of professional status. The development of a professional role in each country is the goal of nursing education. The reforms of nurse education in Sweden (Olsson & Gulberg, 1988), Finland (Katajamaki 1970) and the United Kingdom (UKCC 1986) clearly indicate that changes in the education of nurses are inevitably linked to social policy. This reflects the need to keep nursing competitive in a changing labour market; the need to maintain recruitment and retention levels; the economics of health care; and the need to redress the imbalance between the primary and secondary sectors of the health care system.

In spite of the outward difference of language, nationality and religion, nurses throughout Europe historically have been influenced by each other. In a period of political and economic change in Europe we should be building on these past linkages and learning from each other.

Nursing as a human service

Attempts to identify and compare the tasks performed by nurses throughout the European Region are not only impossible, but a pointless exercise that would merely highlight the differences. A more positive line of enquiry is to focus on the fundamental beliefs that are shared by all and which therefore bind us together.

Nursing is a human service. It is an expression of the concerns individuals have for each other and that societies have for their most vulnerable members. The concept of care of self and others is shared by all members of society and in all countries. These concepts may be defined slightly differently within individual cultures and sub-groups, but they are based on the values and norms concerning the nature of our relationships with each other and ourselves.

Sarvimaki (1988) argued that nursing could be perceived as a form of moral and practical activity. In doing so, Sarvimaki concentrates our attention on the moral values and norms underpinning nursing practice, and the way that practice reflects our rights and duties as individuals and members of society. Nursing, therefore, is an expression of a value according to which it is morally desirable to help others towards something good and a norm which guides the nurse's actions. Nursing care in both the hospital and community settings is an expression of a view of the good life.

The literature reviewed by Sarvimaki to support her argument indicates that this view of nursing as a fundamentally moral act is shared by nurses in different countries. Raatikainen (1989), for example, supports this view of nursing and argues that professional nursing education should be the vehicle for developing strong professional ethics and for enhancing the individual nurse's ability to engage in critical and analytical thinking. Only in this way can nursing overcome its past dependency on routine-based work. Raatikainen argues that a strong belief in the values related to the well-being of individuals engenders in the nurse a feeing of being morally at liberty to make and take responsible and independent decisions.

Throughout Europe there appears to be a growing consensus of nursing opinion that a belief in nursing practice as a morally good activity aids individual nurses to decide how they should relate to others who are unable to look after themselves, or to look after their rights. Such a belief will not remove the dilemmas associated with role extension or expansion. It is however a basis for helping us to decide whether or not the decisions we make in daily practice are in the interest of the common good. Furthermore, it brings to our attention the fact that society will hold us to account for the moral decisions we make and those that we do not make or which we avoid.

Nursing as an organisational role

Nursing care is provided by men and women in their own homes and in the formal health care system. It is, therefore, both a social and organisational role. Within the formal health care organisation, it is predominantly a female occupation. The role of the nurse within the formal health care organisation is based on a gender division of labour in the home and the wider society. Thus the role is influenced by the political, economic and socio-cultural factors of the individual country in which it is practised.

The close proximity of nursing work to that of the medical profession has ensured that the latter has influenced the education and practice of nurses. This control has been exercised through the manipulation of the boundaries between the two roles by the medical profession. In this way, doctors have had a major impact on the job content of nurses and, therefore, the extension of the nurse's role through the delegation of tasks associated with medical diagnosis and treatment. Role expansion as a vehicle for nurses attempting to set their own agenda inevitably creates tensions and conflicts between the social and organisational roles of the doctor and the nurse. Thus the medical profession, directly and indirectly, has determined the degree of both the extension and expansion of the nurse's role. This strategy of autonomy is outlined in Lima Bassto's account of Portuguese nurses' attempts to implement the nursing process (Lima Bassto 1987).

Nursing practice throughout Europe may be viewed as being comprised of three broad categories of activity:

(1)   those activities nurses may perform in their own right;
(2)   those activities which are delegated by doctors and which may be performed without the doctor being present; and
(3)   those activities delegated by the doctors and which may be performed only in their presence.

In terms of role expansion, that is in the development of that aspect of nursing practice which nurses perform in their own right, there will be activities which nurses have taken over from doctors in the past. These activities may now be viewed by nurses as an integral part of their practice and no longer recognised by them as a form of role 'extension'. Furthermore, there may be hidden forms of role expansion that are not necessarily obvious to the nurse. This is more subtle than that exemplified by the taking on of new technical tasks. Taking on responsibilities for clerical tasks associated with medical record keeping, implementing clinical regimes ordered by other health care workers in their absence and assimilating general management tasks into daily practice all constitute role expansion, albeit in a covert form. In the past, nurses have been too willing to take on board the tasks left out by other health care workers under the rationale of providing 'total patient care' and to delegate direct care activities to support workers.

The influence of the medical profession, as role models within a given clinical speciality, on the role of the nurse is highlighted by Dassen *et al.* (1990). In this study of nurses working in intensive care units in the Netherlands, Dassen *et al.* identify the professional socialisation of nurses along traditional gender-specific role patterns. Furthermore, male nurses perceived their jobs in a more medical perspective than did their female colleagues. Thus, the extension of the nurse's role into that of the doctor could be viewed by these nurses as role expansion.

The boundaries between that which constitutes role expansion and that which is role extension are far from clearly defined. Much will depend upon the group's perceptions of its role and the factors shaping nursing practice in a specific clinical setting. Should we, for example, accept Allan's study of intracranial pressure monitoring (1989) in the UK as role extension or expansion? The data presented suggests that both the researcher (Allan) and the subjects considered this technical task as role expansion and therefore a legitimate and integral part of their work.

Both Dassen *et al.* (1990) and Allan (1989) highlight a specific problem for the socialisation of new recruits to nursing. If qualified nurses perceive the medical profession as their role models, they will be attracted to that role, adopt its values and norms, and seek to perform its tasks. Students will wish to model themselves on the qualified nurse. In this way, a cycle develops in which qualified nurses continue to extend their roles as technicians, students are socialised into this role and the fundamentals of nursing care are given to support workers.

The medical profession continues to define nursing and the role of the nurse through their control over job content and the knowledge associated with high technology tasks. Must role expansion always be in terms of developing skills in carrying out tasks integral to role extension?

Over-extending the role of the nurse into those of doctors and technicians opens up the possibility of nursing work being viewed as nothing more than a series of technical tasks. This, in turn, denies the claim that nurses provide a comprehensive service reflecting the clients' demands for nursing care.

In contrast to Allan's (1989) study, Hentinen and Sinkkonen (1985) in Finland report on a programme for developing the nurse's skills and practice in caring for post-myocardial infarction patients. Holistic recovery, these writers argue, does not only depend on the function of the heart and the return of vital functions. The results of this study suggest that planned programmes of change can be implemented in busy hospital wards. Furthermore, these programmes can promote true role expansion through the development of the nurse's knowledge base and problem solving skills, promoting accountability and motivation. This in turn is enhanced through the adoption of a systematic approach to planned nursing care and the organisation of work along the lines of primary nursing (Hentinen & Sinkkonen 1985).

New horizons

Increases in the cost of health care are recorded in all the European countries and all are attempting to control these costs. The ethic of providing everything possible for the individual regardless of cost was achievable when the possibilities were few and relatively inexpensive. The advances in modern medical technology have broadened the scope of health care possibilities, increased demand from the public and created a demand for highly trained and expensive health care professionals, including nurses.

The WHO has identified the progress made in Europe in removing communicable diseases as the major source of ill health and death since the end of the Second World War. This improvement in the health of the population has led to the identification of new targets for health. It is envisaged that the major demands for health care will be related to three main factors:

(1) Heredity – genetic disorders and longevity.
(2) Environment – changing food pathways, occupational health and the impact on the environment of industry.
(3) Accidents – trauma, neoplastic and cerebro-vascular.

It would appear that the increased costs and changing demands for health care throughout the European Region necessitate the targeting of finite resources, including nurses, at the high risk groups, expanding the nurse's role in carrying-out epidemiological studies to monitor existing services, and providing guidelines for meeting future demands.

Throughout the 1970s and 1980s nurses in several European countries have recorded their attempts to change their roles and functions. These changes have focused on the development of a practitioner role for the nurse. The vehicles for such change have been a systematic approach to client-centred care and primary nursing.

Professional journals are publishing an increasing volume of research-based papers describing the attempts made by individuals and groups of nurses to challenge traditional modes of practice. There is, however, little in the way of studies researching the process of nursing across national boundaries. To the best of this writer's knowledge there is only one truly international study of people's demands for nursing care in Europe (Stussi 1985). Given the importance of such a study, it is disappointing to see so little reference to it by nurse scholars and policy makers. The importance of such a study is further emphasised by the current EC Directives on the education of the nurse and the free movement of the nursing workforce within the EC.

In 1977 the International Council of Nurses (ICN) adopted a resolution advocating that nursing should be research-based. Following this, the Regional Officer in the WHO European Regional Office set up the Workshop of European Nurse Researchers (WERN) in 1978. Annual meetings of this group have been held ever since. WERN is now composed of one delegate from each nursing association in Europe in membership of the ICN.

The work of this Group remains largely unknown to the vast majority of nurses. However within the Group the obstacles which result from different backgrounds, culture and language have been overcome and agreements on common goals have been achieved. Glass and Bjorn (1987) record that the initial goals set by WERN relate to the clarification of terminology and the classification of needs for nursing care expressed by populations throughout the European Region. This, in turn led to a WHO study in nursing entitled 'People's Needs for Nursing Care' (Stussi 1985; WHO 1987). This study reinforced the WHO's change in its programme for the nursing services in Europe. These changes centred on a systematic approach to nursing care as an essential element of the education of nurses and the organisation and delivery of care. It could be argued that this change in direction signalled the WHO's support for role expansion, rather than extension, as the means of providing a better quality service, based on the populations' needs for nursing care.

In her introductory speech at the presentation of the multi-national study of peoples' needs for nursing care, Stussi (1985) identified the study's place within the medium-term programme designed by the WHO for the development of nursing in Europe. This medium term programme was composed of four major components: nursing process; nursing education; organisation and management of nursing services; and resource planning. The study into people's needs for nursing care was part of the nursing process component. It was carried out in three successive phases and involved seven nursing research centres in six countries (Belgium, Denmark, Finland, France, Poland and the UK). By 1981 one-third of the Member States (10 European countries) were collaborating in this multi-national study and this included Norway, Greece, Yugoslavia and Czechoslovakia.

The overall purpose of this study (Stussi 1985) was to identify and describe the needs of persons for nursing care, the objectives, the nursing interventions and the outcomes related to those needs, and to establish this data as one source of information which will serve as a database for other projects.

Glass and Bjorn (1987) in their discussion of the findings of this study argue that it demonstrated the difference between nursing and medical care. It also highlighted the leadership required to strengthen nursing in Europe and the changes required in the perception of nursing, its practice and education. These writers also identify the catalytic nature of the study and the continued co-operation between the countries involved to refine the data collection tools and to record nursing and its decision making processes (Stussi 1985; Glass & Bjorn 1987). The adoption of a common framework for nursing practice in this study implies that a common definition of the nurse's role was explicitly and implicitly agreed by the nurses representing the countries involved. This study, therefore, identifies the growing movement in the European Region towards the recognition of nursing as a discipline worthy of study in its own right.

Conclusion

The role of the nurse is changing in response to the political, social and economic factors shaping the diverse health care systems throughout the European Region.

The outward lack of a common agreement on the definition of the role of the nurse and the regulation of nursing practice limits the discussion on role extension and expansion to general issues, rather than focusing on specifics. Role extension is inevitably linked to advances in medical technology, whereas role expansion appears to be more likely to succeed in community based health-orientated services. Both role extension and expansion create tensions between the attempts by nurses to set their own agenda and the factors shaping nursing practice in the clinical areas.

The current literature reflecting nursing practice in mainly the North European countries suggests that nurses adopt both role expansion and extension strategies to develop their professional practice. There is evidence to suggest that nursing education is moving into the higher education sector in most countries. Nursing research is uncovering shared values and norms underpinning the process of nursing. It therefore appears that in spite of outward differences resulting from national boundaries, nurses throughout the Region share common beliefs about the value of nursing as a therapeutic activity in its own right, with an added value over and above the performance of the individual tasks. It is this shared belief that offers us the opportunity to engage in partnerships in practice, education and research.

All changes in nursing require careful scrutiny. When changes in the nurse's job content involve activities classified as role extension, or expansion, the nurse requires critical and analytical thinking skills to make moral decisions about the benefits these changes may bring to individuals and populations. Whatever the future of nursing in Europe it is certain that the dilemmas surrounding role extension and expansion are likely to continue to confront all nurses, regardless of their clinical specialism or country of origin. Closer co-operation between nurses throughout the Region is essential to clarify and validate our beliefs in the value of nursing and its place within the health care system.

In particular, we need more multi-national research into the application of a systematic approach to client-centred care and primary nursing. These vehicles appear to be central to role expansion that is not directly linked to extending the nurse's role into that of other health care workers.

References

Abel-Smith B. (1960) *A History of the Nursing Profession*. Heinemann, London.

Abel-Smith B. (1985) *Eurocare*. Health Service Consultants, Basle.

Allan D. (1989) Intracranial pressure monitoring: a study of nursing practice. *Journal of Advanced Nursing* **14**, 127–131.

Asvall J. E., Jardell J. & Nanda A. (1986) Evaluation of the European strategy for health for all by the year 2000. *Health Policy* **6**, 239–258.

Badouaille M. L. (1972) The staff school of the Red Cross in France 1951–1971. *International Journal of Nursing Studies* **9**, 95–101.

Caspane A. F., Hermans H. E. G. M. & Paelinck J. H. P. (1990) *Competitive Health Care in Europe: Future Prospects*. Dartmouth, Aldershot.

Dassen T. W. N., Nijhuis F. J. N. & Philipsen H. (1990) Male and female nurses in intensive care wards in the Netherlands. *Journal of Advanced Nursing* **15**, 387–393.

Diepeveen-Speekenbrink J. C. M. (1990) Creative international networking towards academic nursing education and research in the Netherlands. *Journal of Advanced Nursing* **15**, 738–743.

Fagermoen M. S. (1984) From apprenticeships to study – the development of nursing education in Norway. *International Journal of Nursing Studies* **21** (3), 165–175.

Glass H. & Bjorn A. (1987) European Work Group. Leadership in Action. In *Clinical Judgement and Decision Making: The Future with Nursing Diagnosis* (eds K. J. Hannah, M. Reimer, W. C. Mills & S. Letourneau). John Wiley and Sons, Chichester.

Grauhan, A. (1970) A survey of the professional activities of former students of the school of nursing, University of Heidelberg. *International Journal of Nursing Studies* **7**, 125–134.

Hentinen M. & Sinkkonen S. (1985) A programme for developing nurses' skills and nursing practice. *Journal of Advanced Nursing* **10**, 405–416.

Katajamaki M. (1970) Facts about nursing in Finland. *International Journal of Nursing Studies* **7**, 249–255.

Kum E. (1972) Nursing in Turkey. *International Journal of Nursing Studies* **9**, 51–58.

Lima Bassto M. (1987) Who's in charge here? They are! In *Clinical Judgement and Decision Making: The Future with Nursing Diagnosis* (eds K. J. Hannah, M. Reimer, W. C. Mills & S. Letourneau). John Wiley and Sons, Chichester.

Milena P. (1972) The development of nursing in the northern part of Yugoslavia. *International Journal of Nursing Studies* **9**, 151–158.

O'Leary G. M. (1972) Nursing in Iceland. *International Journal of Nursing Studies* **9**, 27–32.

OECD (1990) Health care systems in transition. Organisation for Economic Co-operation and Development. *Social Policy Studies* **7**.

Olsson H. M. & Gulberg M. T. (1988) Nursing education and importance of professional status in the nursing role. Expectations and knowledge of the nurse role. *International Journal of Nursing Studies* **25**(4), 287–293.

Paillet-Kelson M. (1992) Nurses' knowledge of the EC. *Nursing Standard* **6**(18), 24–27.

Quinn S. (1982) Nursing education in the countries of the European Community. In *Nursing Education* (ed. M. S. Henderson). Churchill Livingstone, Edinburgh.

Raatikainen R. (1989) Values and ethical principles in Nursing. *Journal of Advanced Nursing* **14**, 92–96.

Rogers J. (1991) The lifeblood of the NHS. *Personnel Management* **June**, 45–49.

Sarvimaki A. (1988) Nursing care as a moral, practical, communicative and creative activity. *Journal of Advanced Nursing* **13**, 462–467.

Stussi E. (1985) Introductory speech to the Presentation of 'People's Needs for Nursing Care – A Multi National Study'. WHO Regional Office for Europe, Vienna, 26 September.

United Kingdom Central Council for Nursing, Midwifery and Health Visiting (1986) *Project 2000: New Preparation for Practice*. UKCC, London.

Uyer G. (1984) Nursing Education in Turkey: past and present. *International Journal of Nursing Studies* **21**(3), 209–219.

World Health Organization (1978) *Alma-Ata 1978: Primary Healthcare*. WHO, Geneva, 2–3.

World Health Organization (1985) *Targets for Health for All*. WHO Regional Office for Europe, Copenhagen.

World Health Organization (1987) *People's Needs for Nursing Care: A European Study*. WHO, Geneva.

World Health Organization (1988) Health services: concepts and information for national planning and management. *Public Health Papers* **67**, 9. WHO, Geneva.

World Health Organization (1989) *Summary Report of the First Meeting of Government Chief Nursing Officers and WHO Collaborating Centres on the Implications of HFA Targets for Nursing and Midwifery* (Linkoping, Sweden, 18–21 October 1989). WHO Regional office for Europe, Copenhagen.

Part II
Areas of Practice

Chapter 7
Specialist and Advanced Nursing and the Scope of Practice

Introduction

The practice of nursing, midwifery and health visiting today is the result of previous historical forces. Many of those forces have resulted in defensive and reactive changes rather than deliberate efforts to develop the potential of nursing practice and broaden the scope for practitioners to be more effective and efficient.

There have been three major forces affecting the context of professional nursing and midwifery practice:

(1) Consumerism and the increasing demands by the public for a more effective, efficient and quality health service. There is a greater awareness and overall demand for better health care and treatment.
(2) The growth of medical science and technology, which has resulted in the rapid and continuing expansion of specialisation and complexity in the delivery of health care. Due to the advancements made in medical technology and treatment people are now surviving extreme illnesses and injuries.
(3) Efforts to professionalise nursing and midwifery and identify the core components, knowledge and skills, which form the basis of clinical practice.

The Department of Health in its document, *A Vision for the Future* (DoH 1993) sets out a new and ambitious strategy for nursing, midwifery and health visiting by outlining targets in five key areas:

- *Quality:* improved care on an individual basis, with outcomes charted and delivery submitted to audit.
- *Accountability:* better care and services by expanding the scope of professional practice.
- *Clinical leadership:* promoting health and new approaches to care through strong leadership, research and supervision.

101

- *Purchasing:* enhancing the efficiency and effectiveness of health care by influencing the commissioning and contracting process.
- *Education:* preparing nurses, midwives and health visitors for the new challenges.

This document, with its emphasis on 12 targets for achievement, markedly contrasts with the more restrictive tone taken in such documents as *The Extending Role of the Nurse* (DHSS 1989; see Appendix V in this volume). Previously limits were placed on the type of duties and tasks nurses and midwives could take on. In addition there was an expectation that special short courses should be taken, and certificates awarded on successful completion, for each new competency. However, such certificates and courses were often not recognised when a nurse or midwife moved from one employer to the next, resulting in professional frustration and duplication of effort.

Since achieving registration and guidance for qualification the profession has been gearing itself towards sustaining nurse generalists who tended to fit the saying 'Jack of all trades, master of none'. When potential developments did arise, for example in aspects of health care relating to nutrition, physiotherapy and activities for daily living, other health care professionals emerged and there was a growth in paramedical and technician support.

The medical profession has appeared to be keen on nurses developing their roles and broadening their education. Unfortunately this enthusiasm was often viewed with suspicion and fear that nurses would extend their practice into medical tasks, leaving their core nursing skills behind as they became mini-doctors. The effects and changes in medical and surgical treatments resulted in the patients' need for a specialist nurse to fill the gap between medical care and nursing. At first these were in areas of care following such physically and emotionally disturbing operations as the removal of part of the body for cancer.

The Joint Board of Clinical Nursing Studies was set up in 1970 to respond to the need for more specialised, advanced post-registration courses for nurses. It was obvious that nurse generalists and teachers of nursing who could keep abreast of the latest discoveries and developments in patient care were fast disappearing.

Professionalisation of nursing was also starting to gain momentum with its acceptance into higher and university education. No longer were nurses being viewed as non-professionals who needed watching because they could not be trusted to manage their own work. There was a shift in the rigid management of nursing which in the past had been preoccupied with organising and administering nurses, making sure that they were doing the tasks expected of them.

The scope of practice in general

The development of specialist and advanced nursing should be seen as going hand in hand with the expansion of the nursing role in general. The UKCC's 1992 document, *The Scope of Professional Practice*, starts by stating that:

> 'Practice takes place in a context of continuing change and development. Such a change and development may result from advances in research leading to improvements in treatment and care, from alterations to the provision of health and social care services, as a result of changes in local policies and as a result of new approaches to professional practice. Practice must, therefore, be sensitive, relevant and responsive to the needs of individual patients and clients and have the capacity to adjust, where and when appropriate to changing circumstances'.

To cope with these developments and responsibilities in practice, the UKCC emphasises that all individual nurses, midwives and health visitors should carefully refer to their own personal experience, education and skill. The answer to what each individual may take on therefore is firmly rooted in what they have previously done and how they have prepared themselves for the future.

There are some professional and legal concerns about the UKCC's document and the possibilities of nurses developing their role and taking on activities previously the domain of other professionals. The document is not suggesting that practitioners should have *carte blanche* to do exactly what they please. There is no agreed list or set number of activities which a practitioner should hold. The achievement and degree of expertise needed in carrying out a required competency is also not covered, leaving the practitioner to guess what level they should reach. By law anyone carrying out a medical task will probably be judged in comparison with a reasonable medical practitioner.

Also, it is difficult to see how standards can be maintained and monitored across the UK if practitioners are not given minimum guidance on what level they should be achieving in their performance. Perhaps the National Nursing and Midwifery Boards in all four countries of the UK could be involved in auditing practitioners' competence.

There is a danger that instead of liberating practitioners there will be extra pressures on them to take on tasks which result in their work becoming more pressurised. It would be an interesting situation if there was a demarcation dispute between practitioner and employer. Who would mediate in disputes over, for example, the extent or length a nurse should go in broadening their practice?

The UKCC makes the point in *The Scope of Professional Practice* that the terms 'extended' or 'extending' roles are, 'no longer suitable since they limit, rather than extend, the parameters of practice'. 'Extension' means stretching out, but from what and to what are nursing and midwifery care being stretched or developed? This is the question which concerns those who see nursing strongly related to a holistic model involving closeness to the patient/client and a type of hands-on approach, of natural healing, understanding and care associated with the arts, rather than medical science.

The luxury of total nursing/midwifery care often gets left behind when economic pressures bring cuts in the health care service. If nursing does not take on new roles and responsibilities it becomes threatened, and is accused of resistance to change and development.

Medical delegation?

There are those, however, who enjoy the challenge of practising nursing in a different setting with the additional demands which the change may make on them. Sometimes what emerges from this direction is an enhanced nursing role or even a nurse specialist, while other times all it results in is a modified version of the physician's assistant or associate. History may show that as nursing lost resources for total patient care, needs assessment and time with patients, so technical nursing came to the fore. As a set of techniques or competencies that relate directly to the delivery of service, the practice of technical nursing offers an exact, unambiguous sort of opportunity to professionalise the work instead of the worker.

To attempt to persuade professionally educated nurses that they should take on medical tasks and function at a lower level in the field of medicine represents an unbelievable human and intellectual waste. What is more, it demonstrates an ignorance of nursing care and an effort to deny society knowledgeable nursing services. Expanding the scope of professional nursing practice means developing the scope of nursing *care*, not moving into medicine or any other field of technical care or manipulation of machinery. Medical knowledge, no matter how relevant to medical practice, is not a substitute for the nursing knowledge that is essential to nursing practice. As Rogers (1970) states:

'The science of nursing is not a summation of facts and principles drawn from other sources; it is a science of synergistic person – unitary person – characterised by an organised conceptual system from which are derived the hypothesised generalisations and unifying principles essential to guide practice.'

The phenomena which nursing seeks to describe, explain and predict differ clearly from the phenomena that are of primary concern to other disciplines. It is nursing knowledge that nurses bring to interdisciplinary case conferences and it is nursing knowledge that adds new dimensions to human needs and health. If the scope of nursing practice is to be developed then it should be for the good of the patient and nursing care. The nursing profession does not exist to take on the delegated tasks of any other profession, particularly medicine. It must determine its own boundaries and be aware of what it is doing when it develops new skills and competencies.

What kind of activity?

Many of the activities commonly attributed within nursing's scope of practice may in fact be attempts to replace nursing practice with non-nursing functions. The following is a list of activities which nurses and midwives could safely develop in their scope of practice.

(1) Assessment of patients' or clients' physical and psychosocial needs.
(2) Sophisticated analysis and identification of nursing/midwifery problems and potential needs.
(3) Expertise in making clinical judgements, nursing diagnoses, prognoses and treatment decisions.
(4) Processing relevant information from clinical situations and human responses to health problems.
(5) Techniques for dealing with nursing and midwifery problems and diagnosis.
(6) Treatment and evaluation strategies based on nursing interventions.
(7) Teaching and educating patients or clients and their friends and relatives.
(8) Developing strategies, linkages between nursing theory and practice.
(9) Nursing tasks associated with nursing judgements and decisions.
(10) Communication and interpersonal skill development.
(11) Activities and behaviour to enhance nurses' credibility and influence in health care decisions.
(12) Information processing, monitoring new machines and nursing equipment.

(13) Consultation and nursing leadership.
(14) Patient advocacy.
(15) Managing and coordinating patient services.

The following activities (although often carried out by nurses/midwives) do little if anything to enhance the scope of nursing/midwifery practice:

(1)   Handed down medical tasks.
(2)   Participating in medical diagnosis.
(3)   Presenting drugs.
(4)   Following physicians' orders.
(5)   Specimen collection and laboratory work.
(6)   Assisting doctors with medical examinations, procedures and investigations.
(7)   Cleaning and maintaining equipment.
(8)   Medical note-taking, recording medical information and statistics and medical audits.
(9)   Carrying out medical treatments.
(10) Performing minor surgical operations and medical techniques.
(11) Managing and coordinating medical clinics and services.
(12) Teaching primarily medical topics.
(13) Disposal of waste.
(14) Assisting with medical ward rounds.
(15) Making tea and coffee.

Specialist and advanced practice

Historical influences

The establishment of specialist and advanced nursing practice probably began with two critical developments in the Nightingale era.

Firstly, there was the establishment of Florence Nightingale's School of Nursing in 1860 and, secondly, the publication of her second version of *Notes on Nursing*, the Library Standard edition, which was directed principally towards professional nurses (Skretkowicz 1992).

Nightingale was responsible for identifying and then linking nursing as a profession with that of a speciality. She principally distinguished between two separate classes of nurses, that is the amateur, hired, domestic servant of Mrs Gamp's notoriety in Charles Dickens' *Martin Chuzzlewit*, and the professionally prepared hospital nurse of St Thomas's fame.

Nursing, like other developing professions, promoted specialisation as a key feature in the process of moving from an occupational group to a profession.

The first type of specialisation to occur in nursing in the United Kingdom was the Nurses' Registration Act 1919, which identified four major specialities: sick children, mental nursing, care of the mentally handicapped, and fever nursing. 'Speciality', like specialist nursing practice, was restricted to knowledge and skills associated with a particular medical condition or disease.

Due to the lack of formal educational courses and an absence of research, it is very difficult to say if these early nurses who specialised in this way developed specialist nursing skills or were just good generalists who adapted well to medical task work. It would seem, however, from examining nurse training syllabuses and noting the shortages of post-registration courses in clinical nursing, that up until the late 1960s nurse education was geared towards preparing and sustaining nurse generalists in limited functional specialities. White (1977) criticised this position when she wrote:

'As a profession we expect ourselves to know everything and if we continue to feel that the general trained nurse must know it all, we shall continue to be a profession which is broadly based in knowledge, but sadly lacking in depth.'

Specialisation infers a narrowing of the range of work to be done, and an increase in the depth of knowledge and skill. In clinical nursing terms it was not until the 1970s that major moves began to happen with regard to clinical specialisation and advanced nursing practice. It is interesting to note that apart from some broad specialisation referred to earlier, the first movements in specialisation in nursing took place not along clinical lines but along what is referred to as, 'functional specialities' such as administration, teaching and planning (Kohnke 1978).

Referring to the 1940s and 1950s Smoyak (1976) points out that most trained nurses' educational teaching was focused away from developing clinical nursing practice but geared towards task-fulfilment, administration and supervision.

One possible reason for this was that nurses were not seen as accountable professionals but individuals who had to be closely supervised and monitored. This position was not helped when the report of the Salmon Committee (DHSS 1966) introduced a hierarchical nursing management structure into UK nursing.

In other countries such as the United States of America, the development of clinical specialisation in nursing has been, in more recent times, closely linked with university education. It appears that ideas were being put into practice with regard to a clinical nursing specialist educated to Masters degree level in the late 1940s. The National League for Nursing (USA) in 1952 supported the concept of a specially prepared nurse clinician when it said: 'The Baccalaureate programme should prepare the nurse for general professional nursing, the Masters programme for specialisation'.

According to the American Nurses' Association (1980) specialisation in nursing is currently well established and is indicative of the advancement of the nursing profession. Sparacino *et al.* (1990, pp. 3–9) further confirm that the clinical nurse specialist role is clearly defined with respect to Masters degree preparation and scope of practice. There is a core content of educational preparation and practice standards which seem to attract and retain highly committed professional nurses who are now demonstrating how effective and valuable the role is.

In the UK there have been four main influences in the move towards identifying clinical nursing specialisation and advanced practice. These can be divided into:

(1) Specialist hospital and health care influence
(2) The Manchester School
(3) The Royal College of Nursing
(4) Political and Professional regulatory influences (Castledine 1991).

Specialist hospital and health care influence

As medicine began to specialise in treatments and technological interventions there was also a need for the nurses role to respond effectively. In some cases this involved nurses taking on skills originally the domain of doctors. On other occasions it was the development of new skills to cope with new patient problems.

The Royal Marsden Hospital was one of the leading specialist hospitals which encouraged its senior nurses to develop their roles and become clinical nurse specialists. Other specialist and non-specialist hospitals followed this example and soon there was a proliferation of nurse specialists working in such areas as stoma care, infection control, diabetes, intensive care, and behavioural therapy.

Many of these specialist nurses were not necessarily developing clinical nursing practice but were responding to the need for a technically competent person to carry out a paramedical procedure. There were those, however, who argued that not only did they take on and improve medical procedures but they incorporated and promoted their nursing care role.

The Manchester School

Experiments to develop nursing practice became a feature of both academic and hospital initiatives in Manchester. First of all there was the Biddulph (1976) experiment in which three senior nursing officers were encouraged to develop their roles as clinical specialists in psychiatric liaison, orthopaedics and neurosurgical nursing.

Secondly, there was the influence of the Department of Nursing at the University which pioneered such developments as nursing process, nursing models, nursing curriculum, joint appointments and a Masters degree in clinical nursing. It was former students of Manchester (e.g. Pearson 1983; Wright 1991) who further influenced the progress of clinical nursing.

The Royal College of Nursing

Over the past 20 years the Royal College of Nursing (RCN) has promoted the importance of a clinical career structure for nurses. It organised a seminar on the subject of the Clinical Nurse Consultant at Leeds Castle in Kent. The result of those discussions was the first publication of its kind, called *New Horizons in Clinical Nursing* (RCN 1975).

Following this, the RCN Association of Nursing Practice and other special interest groups, including one for advanced practitioners, lobbied for the recognition of advanced nursing practice. The RCN Daphne Heald Research Unit also carried out a study which showed the value of specialist nurses.

Professional and Regulatory Influences

There were a number of government sponsored reports which supported the role of clinical nurses and the Department of Health explored possible ways in which specialist nurses could be recognised.

The Royal Commission on the National Health Service (DHSS 1979) pressed for a better clinical career structure and for the development of increased responsibility for clinical decision making by nurses.

Following the foundation of the United Kingdom Central Council for Nurses, Midwives and Health Visitors in 1979, it seemed that the support for clinical nursing developments gained momentum. The publication of *The Code of Conduct* (UKCC 1983), *Exercising Accountability* (UKCC 1989) and *The Scope of Professional Practice* (UKCC 1992) laid the foundations for the 1993 Post-Registration Education and Practice Project (PREPP) proposals for post-registration nursing (UKCC 1990).

Specialist and advanced nursing practice today

For the first time ever in the UK there is now a formal proposal for a recognised definition of post-registration nursing education and practice. Primary practice relates to the period in which the nurse or midwife is able, following a period of support and preceptorship immediately following registration, to accept responsibility with added confidence and competence.

It is acknowledged that pre-registration education and experience within primary practice are not enough to meet the demands of specialist health care. There is a need for specialist post-registration nursing education and clinical career development.

Specialist nursing practice is defined by the UKCC as:

'Practice for which the nurse is required to possess additional knowledge and skill in order to exercise a higher level of clinical judgment and discretion in clinical care and to provide expert clinical care and leadership, teaching and support to others.'

The Council goes on to stress that there is a major difference between practising in primary practice within a 'speciality' and being prepared by a formal educational programme to practise as a 'specialist'. A specialist nursing practitioner is 'a registered nursing practitioner, who has undertaken specific additional preparation to an agreed Council standard, in order to meet specific patient client, and community need' (UKCC 1993).

In nursing carried out primarily in institutions, areas of specialist nursing practice can be grouped into three broad areas according to the nature of nursing intervention.

(1) Critical care nursing, which includes such specialities as intensive care emergency nursing.
(2) Acute care nursing, which encompasses such areas as acute medical/surgical and child and adolescent psychiatry.
(3) Continuing care nursing, which is concerned with among other things the promotion of self-care and rehabilitation, e.g. behavioural psychotherapy nursing, palliative care nursing, nursing the elderly and spinal injury nursing.

In community nursing there is a move to develop specialist nurses and health visitors in the following areas:

(1) Nursing care of adults, e.g. district nurses and practice nurses.

(2) Nursing care of children, e.g. school and paediatric nurses.

(3) Nursing care of the mentally ill.

(4) Nursing care of the mentally handicapped.

(5) Nursing care of employees within the work place, e.g. occupational health nurses.

(6) Nursing contribution to the promotion of community health, child protection and health maintenance, e.g. health visitors.

It is proposed to have a wide range of modular educational programmes, approved by the Council and set at first degree level to meet the needs of specialist nurses.

The UKCC goes on to describe advanced nursing practice as that area of responsibility involving clinical management, leadership, standard setting, quality assurance, audit, practice development and research. Although the UKCC does not give us a definition of 'an advanced nursing practitioner' it is obvious that they see such a person with higher knowledge and skills than a specialist nursing practitioner. Such an individual should be able to provide expert clinical care, clinical leadership, management, teaching, supervision and support.

Advanced practitioners will probably be prepared in future at Masters degree level in their appropriate nursing subject. They should also be primarily the ones who are concerned with adjusting and pushing forward the boundaries of nursing practice, pioneering and developing nursing care in response to patient/client needs and health service demands. For many a critical element of their work will be in evaluation and research.

Nurse practitioners

The UKCC states in the final report on PREPP (UKCC 1993) that it does not recognise the term 'nurse practitioner', as all nurses are practitioners in their own right. There have been several experiments with nurses using the title 'nurse practitioner' (Stilwell 1987). In many cases the term is used to denote a nurse taking on more technical and medically related tasks.

For the sake of preserving and integrating the 'nursing' perspective in such roles, it would seem more sensible to call all such practitioners 'specialist nursing practitioners'. This would also encourage a united approach and an approved standard of integrating certain medical/ technical roles with nursing. It would further avoid fragmentation and the development of a separate specialist nursing group.

Conclusion

Specialist and advanced nursing practice have at long last been recognised in the UK. The UKCC has proposed that there are three areas of nursing practice: primary, specialist and advanced. Each of these three areas requires specific nursing knowledge and skills. The Council will set the standards of education for these three areas but it is acknowledged that they will be at a minimum of Diploma, and first degree level.

This is somewhat different from the situation of clinical specialisation in other countries, particularly North America. For example, in the USA following registration a nurse who wants to develop her clinical career will enter at graduate level and will only be called a clinical nurse specialist following completion of a Masters or Doctorate degree in specialist nursing practice.

Although the situation is different in both countries there is some general agreement about the need for continuing higher education for clinical nursing. While the post-registration specialist nursing role is widely accepted in the United States there is still much work to be done in the UK to justify the UKCC proposals. Those nurses who are developing and practising in specialist and advanced practice will need to evaluate their contribution and value very carefully. Society has yet to fully recognise what nursing's contribution to health care in the 1990s really is. There is still a need to be persuaded that further nursing education and competency development will be an advantage and of value to patients/clients.

Nursing in the UK is on the threshold of a critical change, the answer to which is an expansion in role, of which investment in post-registration education and practice is a crucial element.

References

American Nurses' Association (1980) *Nursing: A social policy statement.* American Nurses' Association, Kansas City.

Biddulph C. (1976) The clinical specialist. In *Nurses & Health Care* (ed. E. Lucas). King Edward's Hospital Fund, London.

Castledine G. (1991) The advanced nurse practitioner, Part I. *Nursing Standard* 5(43), 34–36.

Department of Health & Social Security (1966) *Salmon Report of the Committee on the Senior Nursing Staff Structure.* DHSS, London.

Department of Health & Social Security (1979) *Report of the Royal Commission in the National Health Service.* DHSS, London.

Department of Health & Social Security (1989) *The extending role of the nurse.* Health Circular P1/CMO (89)7 PL/CBO(89)10. DHSS, London.

Department of Health (1993) *A Vision for the Future*. DoH, National Health Service Management Executive, London.

Kohnke M. (1978) The case for consultation. In *Nursing Designs for Professional Practice*. Wiley & Sons, New York.

National League for Nursing (1952) *Report of the Work Conference on Graduate Nurse Education*. Nursing Education Division (Sept 8–11) (mimeographed). NLN, New York.

Pearson A. (1983) *The Clinical Nursing Unit*. Heinemann, London.

Rogers M. E. (1970) *An Introduction to the Theoretical Basis of Nursing*. F A Davies, Philadelphia.

Royal College of Nursing (1975) *New Horizons in Clinical Nursing*. RCN, London.

Skretkowicz V. (1992) *Florence Nightingale's Notes on Nursing*. Scutari Press, London.

Smoyak S. (1976) Specialisation in nursing: from then to now. *Nursing Outlok* **24**(11), 676–681.

Sparacino P. S. A., Cooper D. M. & Minarik P. (1990) *The Clinical Nurse Specialist*. Appleton and Lang, Norwalk, Connecticut.

Stilwell B. (1987) A nurse practitioner in general practice: working style and pattern of consultation. *Journal of Royal College of General Practitioners* **37**, 154–157.

United Kingdom Central Council for Nursing, Midwifery and Health Visiting (1983) *Code of Professional Conduct for the Nurse, Midwife and Health Visitor*. UKCC, London.

United Kingdom Central Council for Nursing, Midwifery and Health Visiting (1989) *Exercising Accountability*. UKCC, London.

United Kingdom Central Council for Nursing, Midwifery and Health Visiting (1990) *Report of the Post-Registration Education & Practice Project* (PREPP). UKCC, London.

United Kingdom Central Council for Nursing, Midwifery and Health Visiting (1992) *The Scope of Professional Practice*. UKCC, London.

United Kingdom Central Council for Nursing, Midwifery and Health Visiting (1993) *Final Report on The Future of Professional Education and Practice*. UKCC, London.

White R. (1977) Mature or matutinal. *Nursing Mirror* **144**(16), 41.

Wright S. (1991) The nurse as a consultant. *Nursing Standard* **5**(20), 30–34.

Chapter 8
The Expanded Role of the Nurse in Intensive Care: A National Survey

Introduction

For many years there has been discussion about the 'extended role' of the nurse with very little clarity about what 'extension' means. The Department of Health and Social Security in its health circular HC(77)22 explained that in relation to the role of the doctor 'the clinical nursing role ... may be extended in two ways, viz. by delegation by the doctor and in response to an emergency' (DHSS 1977). In conjunction with this circular, the Chief Medical Officer (CMO) and Chief Nursing Officer (CNO) wrote a joint letter which pointed out:

> 'If delegation of a particular procedure ... is found to be desirable it is likely that the necessary training will in due course be included in basic or post-basic training and that the procedure will become an integral part of the nurse's role' (Yellowkeys & Friend 1977).

In tro This statement assumes that, as Rowden says, 'In the context of nursing, an extended role is one which is not covered in basic training for the register' (Rowden 1987). But in today's world of professional nursing such an approach has been challenged. The Welsh National Board, for example, in its discussion paper on the subject seems to have been in disagreement with the views of the authors previously cited. The Board regarded the concept of the 'extended role' given by Rowden and others as being:

> 'in direct opposition to any claim that nursing is an independent profession and that nurses are responsible and accountable for their practice: members of most professions recognise the need to modify and adapt their practice as new techniques become available, and one of the hallmarks of professional practice is the ability and willingness to continue to learn new skills' (Welsh National Board 1990).

Indeed, for some time there were deep divisions between different health care professionals in their perception of the changing role of the nurse. The ideas in the UKCC's publication, *The Scope of Professional Practice* (1992) appear to be very much in line with the Welsh National Board document of 2 years earlier. It appears that the straitjacket of piecemeal certification is finally being lifted from our profession. Of course, there are those who are afraid that nurses are being stripped of the only protection they had. The Department of Health in a recent document (Jarvis *et al.* 1992) rescinded all previous advice to health authorities on the 'extended role'.

Over the years there has been considerable discussion about the nature of the extended role and the tasks that may or may not be undertaken by nurses, and some of this is reviewed by Bridgit Dimond in Chapter 4. Intensive Care is an area in which the problem is particularly important, given the range of technical tasks which practitioners may be asked to undertake. However, the tasks and procedures carried out by intensive care nurses vary from one unit to another, depending on the nature of the unit and any local policies. The survey described here was therefore carried out to find out what tasks nurses in this area are performing and what their views are of their role and changes to it.

Method

A questionnaire survey was used to achieve comprehensive coverage of the UK. The questionnaire used both open and closed questions, the latter using both 'Yes/No' and multiple choice responses. A total of 1440 questionnaires were sent to 288 general intensive care units (ICUs) in England, Scotland, Northern Ireland, Wales, the Channel Islands and the Isle of Man; five questionnaires were sent to each unit.

The questionnaires were sent to the senior nurse manager for each ICU together with a list of random numbers. The nurse manager was asked to number all the staff in accordance with their position on the duty roster i.e. first on the roster, No. 1, twelfth on the roster No. 12, down to the last. Then using the list of random numbers the manager was asked to choose the first five random numbers which corresponded to numbers on the roster sheet and distribute the five questionnaires to those five staff members. The staff members were also given a Freepost envelope which was addressed to the research team at The Hammersmith Hospital. By the closing date, 885 questionnaires had been received. This represents a response rate of 61.45%.

Results

Procedures, grades and experience

The first half of the questionnaire listed all the procedures which in the opinion of the researchers, from their experiences in a number of different ICUs, were generally regarded as 'extending' the nurse's role.[1] The respondents were asked to say whether they undertook these procedures, and a variety of reasons for doing so and for not doing so were available as responses. Respondents were then asked whether they thought the procedure listed should be regarded as standard practice for ICU nurses.

Table 8.1 presents a list of the procedures together with the percentage of respondents who are currently carrying out those procedures and the percentage who agreed a procedure should be standard practice.

Section Two of the questionnaire collected data relating to the

Table 8.1   Responses to questions about (a) which procedures are undertaken and (b) which should be regarded as standard practice.*

Procedure	(a)	(b)
Intravenous drug administration	88.10	70.20
Arterial-line sampling	80.00	76.60
Hyperinflation of adults	72.80	77.90
Twelve-lead ECG	68.20	81.50
Extubation	62.20	63.60
Drug infusion titration	58.80	59.70
Blood gas determination	57.80	65.80
Wedging of PA balloon	45.80	40.70
Swan-Ganz catheter removal	43.70	45.20
Hyperinflation of children	42.10	53.20
Alteration of FiO_2 (WPMC)	33.80	44.00
Defibrillation	33.60	36.30
Venepuncture	27.10	43.60
Alteration of ventilation mode (WPMC)	26.10	32.00
Alteration of respiratory rate (WPMC)	21.70	32.40
Alteration of tidal volume (WPMC)	20.80	31.50
Cardiac output estimation	18.90	26.50
Intubation	5.50	12.50
Venous cannulation	2.90	27.70
Arteriopuncture	2.60	9.70

* No. of respondents = 885.   WPMC = without prior medical consultation.
Figures are percentages. FiO_2 = fractional inspired oxygen.
                                          PA = pulmonary artery.

Table 8.2 Defibrillation.

Grade	Percentage of respondents who were trained to carry out defibrillation and did so
C	10.0
D	14.7
E	26.5
F	46.0
G	56.5
H	65.6

There was a highly significant relationship between seniority of grade and whether or not the respondent carried out defibrillation ($n=289$, $P < 0.001$).

respondents themselves: employment grade, gender, health authority region, length of time in ICU and post-basic experience.

The responses to Section One can obviously be cross-related to grade, experience and post-basic course. If this is done for the list of procedures and whether or not they are undertaken by staff, it is evident that (as one would expect) the more experienced, the more highly graded and the more highly trained a staff member is, the more extended procedures they take on. One interesting example of this was the procedure of defibrillation. When broken down by grade we obtained the data given in Table 8.2.

Some results were perhaps a little unexpected, such as those for Swan-Ganz catheter removal and pulmonary wedge pressure monitoring (Table 8.3).

If we consider the respondents' views on whether or not the procedures should form part of an ICU nurse's standard role or be considered

Table 8.3 Experience and selected procedures: (a) percentage of respondents who were trained to carry out Swan-Ganz removal and did so; (b) percentage of respondents who were trained to carry out wedge pressure recording and did so.

Time in ICU	(a)	(b)
0–3 years	33.0	35.5
4–6 years	55.4	55.8
7–9 years	52.8	52.4
10 years or more	43.1	48.7
	($P < 0.001$)	($P < 0.001$)
	($n=375$)	($n=394$)

as extending that role, we can again break the responses down by grade, length of time in ICU and post-basic course. Analysis suggests that staff with greater experience in ICU, or who had attended a post-basic course, were significantly more likely to consider procedures a part of the standard role of the ICU nurse. For example, 5.1% of staff with 4–6 years experience thought intubation should be standard practice, whereas 15.7% of those with 7–9 years and 21.1% of those with 10 or more years experience were of this opinion ($P < 0.001$).

Staff who had completed post-basic courses were more likely than those who had not to consider technical tasks part of the standard role. For example, of those who had not attended an ICU course 36.6% thought pulmonary wedge pressure measurement should be standard practice, whereas of those who had attended a course 44.8% thought this should be the case.

Some of the respondents thought our question about whether they were male or female was sexist. Our reason for posing this question was to examine the common assertion which is made in ICU circles that the male staff are very keen on ICU technology and associated technical procedures. Of the listed procedures there were only five which showed a statistically significant difference in responses from male and female nursing staff. These were arteriopuncture, venous cannulation, arterial line sampling, intubation and cardiac output measurement. Closer inspection shows that the main difference between the responses is that the number of male staff without specific training who are undertaking these procedures is higher than the number of female staff who undertake these procedures without being trained to do so. Several explanations are possible. For instance, are the male staff more likely to be asked to do these tasks or are they more independent in their decision-making or perhaps more foolhardy or prepared to take risks?

Responses to Section Two questions ($n = 883$) are listed below:

Grades:

C Grade	1.1%
D Grade	22.7%
E Grade	39.7%
F Grade	14.4%
G Grade	18.4%
H Grade	3.7%

Sex:

Male	13.0%
Female	87.0%

Shifts:		*Experience in ICU:*	
Days only	15.4%	0–3 years	41.1%
Nights only	7.3%	4–6 years	27.0%
Days and Nights	77.4%	7–9 years	14.5%
		10 or more years	17.4%

Qualifications:

No post-basic course	49.7%
RGN with ENB ICU course	38.0%
EN with ENB ICU course	2.6%
Other ENB course	3.8%
Non-ENB course	5.9%

The percentages of respondents working in the different health authority regions are:

Northern	6.2%	Oxford	3.9%
Yorkshire	5.4%	South Western	5.7%
Trent	7.9%	West Midlands	7.9%
East Anglia	5.5%	Mersey	3.3%
North West Thames	6.7%	North Western	7.7%
North East Thames	4.4%	Wales	5.5%
South East Thames	8.3%	Scotland	5.7%
South West Thames	3.7%	Northern Ireland	4.0%
Wessex	5.2%	Isle of Man & Channel Is.	2.9%

The responses to Section 2 of the questionnaire give a snapshot of the current population of ICU staff in the UK. The survey suggests that there is a considerable body of experience within this population, as although the largest single category, at 41.1%, is from 0–3 years working in ICU, almost 60% had worked there for more than three years, and 32% for more than six years. It is disappointing that almost exactly half the sample (49.7%) had no post-basic qualification: it would seem that 8% had worked in ICU for more than three years but had not had the opportunity to attend a post-basic course. With regard to grade mix, more than three quarters of the sample were at E grade or above. It would be interesting to repeat the survey in a few years time, to see whether the PREP recommendations and the continuing implementation of the NHS reforms result in any changes in grade or skill mix.

Staffing and patient care

Section Three questions were designed to give an insight into the extension of ICU nurses' role in relation to patient care, staffing in the ICU and some professional issues. It was encouraging to see that 69% of respondents felt *encouraged* to extend their nursing role, most of them citing senior colleagues or themselves as the motivation behind the extension. On this point there was no significant difference across gender, experience, qualifications or grades.

One question aimed to ascertain whether nurses thought they were under pressure to 'extend' their role. In fact, 82.9% of respondents thought not, but 17.0% said that they had been pressurised. One of the respondents reported 'I was ordered to cannulate a patient's chest by a doctor, as the patient had a tension pneumothorax'. Among the procedures the pressurised respondents were asked to take on, haemofiltration was cited by a few. Also mentioned were intubation, removal of Swan-Ganz catheter, wedging of pulmonary artery balloon, setting up of an epidural and alteration of ventilator settings. Some staff said they only felt pressurised when there was a staff shortage or high workload.

One sister in the Yorkshire region admitted the following: 'G grade sisters are expected to gain experience in death certification. When on duty they are expected to attend wards, not ICU, to confirm the death of patients. This is to save staff from waking the on-call medical staff'.

Of those staff who answered in the negative some made a comment to this effect: 'Doctors sometimes pressure us, as professionals we should be able to stand up for the limits of our knowledge'. Others were more forthright and made statements such as, 'I always refuse – unless supervised', 'if pressured I quote the UKCC code of professional conduct!'.

It would seem that men in ICUs are significantly more likely than women to risk carrying out a procedure for which they had not been trained. When asked 'Are there circumstances in which you would take on an extended role procedure for which you were not certificated or trained?' the result for the total sample was 'Yes' 37.6%, 'No' 49.6%. However, 46% of the men in the sample responded 'Yes' while only 36% of the women did so ($P < 0.01$).

Some of the respondents' comments relating to this question were that they would undertake a procedure for which they were untrained, 'If a patient's life was at risk', 'If there was only a locum doctor on call', and 'If we were understaffed'. One nurse commented that 'The UKCC code of professional conduct puts us in a no-win situation'. Presumably this person was referring to the apparently widely held belief that if a nurse does not undertake a procedure in a life-threatening situation and the patient dies she could be seen as having been negligent, but if she tries to assist the patient and the patient still dies she could be regarded as acting outside her competence.

Some of the procedures these respondents felt they would take on were as follows:

- *Intubation.* Two E grade staff commented 'I would attempt intubation if there was no anaesthetist present'.
- *Defibrillation in the event of cardiac arrest.* 'In VF I would defibrillate as time is an important factor'.
- *Cannulation* 'Insertion of a cannula into the intercostal space when threatened by tension pneumothorax and no medical assistance available'.

Those who would not undertake procedures for which they were untrained commented: 'I'm not prepared to risk my registration'; 'Such circumstances should never arise on an ICU'; 'No, because it might seem the right thing to do, but afterwards the hierarchy would cause so many problems it is not worth it'; 'If there is going to be a delay, in treatment in an emergency situation, longer than thirty seconds then the unit should have a hard look at its policies – untrained hands can be very dangerous!'; 'My Health Authority would not back me up if I carried out a procedure I was not covered to do'.

Comments from the 11.8% of the responses to this question which fell in the 'don't know' category were, 'depends on medical support available', 'if there was a chance to save a life'.

We found that around 77.1% of staff felt that extending one's role was for the patient's benefit as opposed to that of the doctor or nurse. However, 13.9% felt that the extension of their role was for the benefit of doctors and 4.6% felt it was for the benefit of nurses themselves. Regarding patient benefits, comments were: 'Benefits all concerned as procedures done on time'; 'Much more holistic approach to patient care'; 'drugs etc., as well as emergency procedures such as defibrillation can be carried out straight away'. Comments assuming that doctors were the beneficiaries included, 'doctors only want to off-load their responsibilities onto nursing staff', 'many doctors would have more time to do more important things!'.

The results showed that 88.3% of respondents felt that extension of role had a beneficial effect on the way in which they provided total patient care. Common comments were that being able to carry out different procedures enhanced continuity of care and facilitated better care planning. However, of the 2% who felt that role extension was *harmful* to patient care, two comments were, 'some nurses may neglect less glamorous roles and aspects of care in favour of hi-tech roles' and 'some nurses end up nursing the equipment and not the patient in the bed'. Another comment was, 'what is the point of role extension if it is not going to be of benefit', and one of the 7.1% of staff who felt that extending one's role had no significant effect on patient care said, 'there should be no difference to the standard of care'.

The next question asked nursing staff to put themselves in the patient's position. It asked whether they would prefer as a patient to be in a unit in which nurses were encouraged to extend their role or not; 83.1% preferred the former. However, 11.4% would rather have nurses who had not extended their role and 3.4% did not know. Two of the comments by those who felt happier with nurses who had extended their role were as follows: 'I would rather have a competent trained nurse to look after me than a junior doctor with little experience'; and '[a unit which promotes role extension] builds up [patient's] confidence and trust in the carer'.

Even though the majority preferred a unit where extension of the role was promoted, there were some reservations, and these were mainly concerned with the level of training, experience and knowledge: 'as long as adequate training was given and regular assessments'; 'as long as good training facilities were available'. Some of those with the opposing view felt that 'often role extension interferes with nursing care' and 'many patients would be unaware of limitations of nurses by their Health Authority, and are passive to therapy'. Those who had no preference felt that as long as the standard of care was high it was of little consequence who did what. There was no significant difference in responses across gender, grade, experience or training.

In the next question respondents were asked whether they felt that role extension had a beneficial effect, harmful effect, or no significant effect on the *control* which patients had over their own situation. Only 1.1% of staff felt that the effect was harmful, but there was an almost even split between those who thought that role extension had a beneficial effect and those who thought it had no significant effect (45.2% and 42.4% respectively; 11.4% did not know). The comments associated with those who considered role extension beneficial to patients' control were: 'improves the situation as better relationships made with nurses . . . many patients communicate more freely with the nurses'; 'Patients can be assured of prompt action if a problem arises'. Those who felt there was no significance said things like: 'Patients generally do not mind who does what, especially in ICU'. One comment received for this question was: 'Too many nurses spend a lot of time trying to be mini-doctors'. Again, there was no significant difference in responses across gender, grade, experience or training.

Professional issues

One question asked whether or not role extension had an effect on the inter-professional relationships between nurses and between nurses and other health care professionals: 62.3% of respondents considered extension was a strengthening influence and only 6.1% thought it divisive; 12.4% felt it had no significant effect and 19.2% of the staff did not know. As can be seen, the majority of respondents felt that role extension would strengthen relationships, and two of the reasons given were: 'Doctor–nurse relationship would be more equal'; 'A nurse with a good insight into patients' condition/progress can ensure effective communication with other health care professionals'. Comments from those who felt relationships would become weaker were: 'Nurses may be taken advantage of'; 'There is an attitude from nurses in areas other than ICU, that ICU staff are different, I think due to the fact that some of them have never worked in ICU'. There was also the comment that, 'some nurses in other areas may become against critical care nurses, assuming that ICU nurses regard themselves as the elite of the profession'.

Nursing staff often comment that they are busy or have insufficient staff for their workload, so we wanted to examine the perception of the effect of role extension on workload: whether extension increases stress, decreases stress or makes no difference. It turned out that 40.9% felt that it increased stress, 26.3% that it decreased stress, 29.1% said it made no difference and 3.8% did not know.

There were quite a different number of comments in relation to this question. Those who thought extending their role would increase stress gave the following reasons: 'If the unit is short staffed and only a few nurses can carry out a particular procedure, they spend all their time doing that'; 'currently I am on a unit which is very short-staffed and I feel that I couldn't take on any more tasks ... I would be happy if there were sufficient staff and support'; 'the stress is increased by not being able to take on extended procedures'.

However, most of the comments received related to the 26.3% of staff who felt that extending the role reduced their stress. Many of the respondents agreed that being able to carry out extended procedures allowed staff to plan their work much more effectively. Typical of comments were: 'it is very stressful waiting for bloods, etc., so much less so to be able to do them yourself, get the results back so decisions can be made'; 'I don't have to take a senior nurse away from his/her patient to do a procedure I could easily do for myself'; 'don't have to argue with doctors to come and do something'; 'decrease stress, increase job satisfaction and feeling of self-worth'.

Some comments suggested that role extension could either increase or decrease stress, depending on the circumstances. For example one respondent said 'Increases stress if abused therefore nurses must not be afraid to refuse to carry out role extension if too busy or not appropriate', and another said 'One has to be assertive and be able to withdraw extended role when workload too great'. Perceptions of stress varied with post-basic course status. Of those without a post-basic qualification ($n = 420$) 21.7% felt that role extension reduced stress, while 30.1% of those who held an ICU-relevant qualification ($n = 419$) thought this. Of those without an ICU qualification 41.7% thought extended role activities might increase stress, while 40.8% of those with a post-basic course held this view. The relationship between stress and post-basic qualification was significant (Chi Square, $P < 0.05$).

More technicians?

In the intensive care field one sometimes hears talk of introducing technicians to take over some of the duties presently performed by nursing staff. We know that at interview for intensive care nursing posts it is not unusual for a member of the panel to ask why an expensive nurse should be employed when a technician can do the job just as well. We asked the question, 'What effect do you think role extension would have on the introduction of technicians into ICUs?'.

The responses were quite varied with no real majority showing through: 18.4% of respondents felt that role extension would speed up the introduction of technicians into ICUs, 32.0% thought it would slow it down, 16.5% thought there would be no difference and 33.1% did not know. The comments, however, did seem to fall into two main categories. Some respondents maintained that nursing staff are already doing, or are in the best position to do, extended procedures which otherwise might fall to technicians: 'why employ specialists when you can have a jack-of-all-trades'; 'if we do it why employ paramedics at extra cost'; 'if we role-extend then technicians won't be needed'; 'with nurses taking on more extended procedures there is no need for technicians to creep into ICUs'.

Others maintained that technicians should be employed so as to allow nursing staff to nurse and not act as technicians: 'Technicians would lessen the need for nurses to extend their role'; 'Technicians are good value in ICU'; 'Technicians can take on a role that will leave more time for the nurse to do other procedures and care'. One respondent complained that the introduction of technicians to carry out various procedures in her unit now limits the nursing staff's experience in these areas.

This question showed a significant difference when the responses were related to other variables. It seems that the longer staff have been in ICU (with 4–6 year range being the exception) the more they consider that role extension will speed up the introduction of technicians into ICU: those with 0–3 years experience ($n = 351$), 17.7%; 4–6 years ($n = 227$), 15.4%; 7–9 years ($n = 119$) 21.8%; and those staff with 10 years or more experience 22.3%.

The 'slow down' responses were 33.3%, 31.7%, 31.1% and 29.1% respectively, 'no-effect' responses were very slightly different and 'don't knows' were 37.6%, 32.2%, 27.7% and 28.4% respectively ($P < 0.05$). There was also a significant difference between those staff who held no post-basic ICU qualification and those who did. The main area of difference was that 28.9% of non-course-holders ($n = 415$) felt that role extension would slow down the introduction of technicians into ICUs but 34.6% of the course holders thought so ($n = 422$, $P < 0.01$).

Training and education

Training and education for extended procedures has always been considered vitally important, effective and safe practice being paramount. The shift from 'role extension' to 'role expansion', with the UKCC's 1992 document on the scope of professional practice, only changes the emphasis from a piecemeal to a global approach. At the time of our research we were still thinking largely in terms of training for each procedure.

The questionnaire asked whether or not the training the respondents had received had been adequate or not, and 74% said adequate whilst 23.1% said inadequate, with 2.9% having no training. Some of those who considered the training adequate made the following comments: 'Adequate, but would like to see a more formalised system and regular updating', 'Regular updating and experience is required to maintain standards'.

There were many more comments from those respondents who considered the training, if any, inadequate: 'No "real" training, just hands-on experience and teaching from colleagues'; 'Inadequate, see it – do it – teach it!'; 'No support from my manager'; 'Inadequate, as no regular assessment'.

We also considered the process of re-training when changing jobs to a different hospital, asking if standardisation of procedures nationally or health authority wide was needed or not: 72.3% said nationally and 22.3% said across a health authority, with only 3.8% saying no. Only two comments were received from this last group, both along the lines of: 'I think individual units should draw up their own extended roles, as each unit varies greatly in types of admissions'.

The remainder of the comments were in line with the 94.6% of respondents who are in favour of some type of standardisation, be it nationally or health authority wide: 'A recognised national standard is desperately required which allows a nurse to practise her skills in any health authority without having to acquire a local certificate of competence'; 'Yes, so all the critical care areas have at least some basic core roles'; 'Some should be incorporated with ENB courses, therefore accepted if you have done the course'.

Job satisfaction, autonomy and litigation

Job prospects are always important to nursing staff, especially in an area such as intensive care which has a high turnover of staff: 59.8% of staff said they would be more likely to stay on in a unit which allowed role extension, 36.0% said it made no difference and only 1.7% said they would be less likely to stay (2.5% did not know). There were very few comments associated with this question. Those who did comment were all from the 59.8% of staff who would be more likely to remain in a unit which promoted role extension. Comments included: 'More job satis-faction, increased feeling of self-worth'; 'I don't want to be just a doctor's handmaiden of the '90s'.

The implications for recruitment and retention were further explored in the next question. Respondents were asked, 'When looking for a new post, does having a wide range of procedures available to you in a par-ticular ICU have an effect on whether you would apply for a post there?': 57.1% would be more likely to apply for jobs in units which allowed extension, 34.6% said it made no difference, 2.4% would be less likely to apply and 5.8% did not know.

Again the comments were few and far between for this particular question: 'Having worked in a unit where extended role is available I would feel something is missing if I was in a unit which did not provide role extension'; 'More likely to apply as more interest and more autonomy'; 'Yes, a chance to gain knowledge and skills'; 'Not really considered it'; 'No effect, but might be deciding factor whether to stay'. Again as with the previous question, analysis across variables proved insignificant.

Nurses' decision-making and freedom of action is an issue which was explored in two questions. Staff were firstly asked whether extending their role affected the independence of their decision making: 83.1% felt that role extension gave them greater independence. Only 0.9% felt it gave them less independence, 12.8% considered it as having no effect, and 3.2% did not know. The only comments received were in support of the majority of staff: 'Allows greater independence and freedom, increases feeling of heading towards professional status'; 'Greater independence will make you think about the actions you take much more, and this can only be a good thing'; 'Greater independence will lead to greater motivation'.

Another question asked directly whether or not nurses should be given more independence to decide and act: 31.2% felt the current level was quite satisfactory and 58.7% felt they should be able to do more, while 10.1% did not know.

There were a few comments made in support of the various responses: 'Should be encouraged to take on more decision making but with senior management consent', 'Increased, but only as and when the nurse feels confident to do so and is adequately trained and assessed'. Of those who considered that the level of decision making should remain the same, the comments included: 'There would be no support from doctors in the event of litigation', 'We are not mini doctors', 'There is always the fear of litigation'. Some of the respondents expressed concern as to what the Trust hospitals would allow nurses to undertake, and whether the fear of litigation would be too high a price to pay for allowing nurses more freedom to make decisions.

They were also asked specifically whether or not role extension would have an effect on the likelihood of their encountering litigation arising from their day-to-day professional activities: 70% of the respondents felt that there was a greater likelihood of them encountering litigation as a result of role extension. Only 3.9% felt that extending their role was less likely to result in them becoming involved in litigation, 16.0% considered it would have no effect and 9.4% did not know. It is interesting to note that although 70% of staff felt that litigation would be more likely when extending their role, this does not seem to be decisive in putting them off undertaking extended procedures.

The comments provide some evidence of the confusion surrounding the issues of nurses, the law and subjects like vicarious liability: 'A greater likelihood, so nurses have to be made aware of the legal implications of role extension'; 'A risk worth taking if we wish to become recognised as a true profession'; 'Only when mistakes are made'; 'The more that nurses take on, so does the increased probability of human error'. Some of the 3.9% shown above, who considered it less likely that they would encounter litigation said: 'Not if proper training is given and backup from management'; 'Health Authorities will have to provide the vicarious liability cover of nurses wishing to extend their role'. From the 16.0% who felt it would make no difference the comments were: 'Surely [the risk of litigation] will be no greater than it already is'; 'Hopefully there will be no effect on the prospect of litigation'.

Basic training and certification

As we saw, the extended role was originally conceived by some as taking on tasks not taught in basic training. We asked if the procedures which are currently seen as extending the role (listed by us) should be included in basic training: 57.7% said No and 33.6% said Yes, 5.9% put 'Other' comments in, and 2.8% did not know. Considerably more male staff (47%) thought inclusion in the basic curriculum was warranted compared with female staff (31%) ($n = 846$, $P < 0.01$). 'No' responses were 49.5% and 59% respectively.

Another statistically significant variation was discovered when looking at the responses by length of time in an ICU. It seems the longer staff have been in intensive care the more they consider that the extended procedures should be included in basic training. Of staff who have been in ICU 4–6 years, 28.2% said Yes, for 7–9 years, 30.6% said Yes, and of those staff who had over 10 years experience in ICU, 46% felt that the extended procedures should be taught as part of basic training ($n = 848$, $P < 0.01$).

There were some interesting comments associated with this question: 'Yes, especially intravenous drug administration'; 'Yes, but not to the extent of losing other skills such as conversation!'; 'Yes, those procedures commonly used in general areas, e.g. IV drugs, ECG recording'; 'No, many roles are within specialist areas'; 'No, it should remain the individual's choice to take on extended role or not'; 'No, you have to learn the basic skills of nursing first'; 'It should remain the nurse's choice to extend their role or not, but, not doing so should not affect the chance of improving their career'; 'Many roles are part of everyday work in ICU'; 'Who would teach them? Possibly out-of-touch nurse tutors?'.

One of the key features of *The Scope of Professional Practice* is the removal of the requirement for nurses to be certified as competent to undertake a particular procedure. We asked the staff to consider whether having to be certified to take on an extended procedure contradicted any claim that nursing is an independent profession? The response may be somewhat disheartening in official quarters since only 22.3% of respondents answered Yes: 64.6% evidently have a different view of what constitutes a profession as they answered No (12.4% did not know and 0.7% answered under the 'Other' option). There was a statistically significant difference between the opinion of the sexes in that 40% of the male respondents agreed it contradicted professionalism while only 19% of the female respondents agreed ('No' responses were 50.5% and 67% respectively) ($n = 854$, $P < 0.001$).

Once again this question provoked some very interesting and diverse comments, for example: 'Yes, nursing is not a profession'; 'Yes, completely'; 'No, as long as it is run by nurses and assessed by nurses'; 'No, as long as there is no interference from doctors'; 'No, do not all professionals in whatever field have to be deemed competent?'; 'No, it only makes you proficient in that particular task'; 'No, it surely increases the standards of care'; 'No, if the role is not in basic training then we have to have formal assessment and certification'.

When asked whether or not they thought the system of certification was necessary 87.8% said they felt it was, 7.6% thought not, and 4.7% did not know. The large number who support the certification of the extended role may seem to be out of step with the thinking behind the UKCC *Scope of Professional Practice* document and of other critics of role extension. However it is perhaps not surprising that practitioners, many of whom are comparatively junior and inexperienced, working in an area where technical interventions are proliferating, should seek clear, simple guidance.

The comments associated with this question are diverse: 'Necessary, in case of litigation'; 'Necessary but being certified does not always mean you are competent'; 'Necessary but should be transferable between health authorities'; 'Unnecessary, I have attended three study days for the same procedure in three different health authorities'; 'If trained in critical care nursing, it should not be necessary to be assessed and certified over and over again'. Amongst the 'don't knows' were: 'What system, is there one?'; 'More guidelines needed to clarify what is competence'; 'Certification is often given without adequate training anyway!'.

When relating these responses to the other variables it was apparent that the only statistically significant difference was with grade. It seems that F grade staff consider the certification to be most important, with 93.4% of them saying it is necessary, compared with 85.8% of D, 86.7% of E and 88.5% of G and H grades ($n = 849$, $P < 0.05$).

Conclusion

Our research shows what proportion of intensive care nurses perform specific kinds of procedures often regarded as 'extended' and relates this to employment grade, gender, Health Authority Region, length of time in ICU and post-basic education. It suggests that in intensive care nursing at least: most nurses *inter alia* want to extend their role and feel encouraged to do so; they are quite prepared to reconceive many 'extended' procedures as standard; they believe extension would give them greater job satisfaction; they believe that it is better for patients; but they believe certification is necessary and that some kind of national standardisation would be helpful; and they believe extension increases risks of litigation.

The most general conclusion one might reach, tentatively of course, is that ICU nurses appear to wish to extend (or even expand) their role, but see dangers in doing so and thus wish to hang on to formal structures such as certification and standardisation.

Acknowledgements

This research began its life as an assignment we undertook while attending the ENB100 (General Intensive Care Nursing) course at The Hammersmith Hospital in London. With the help of a research grant from Hammersmith and Queen Charlotte's Special Health Authority, for which we are grateful, we were able to treat this assignment as a pilot study and move on to a national survey under the supervision of Geoffrey Hunt, then Director of the National Centre for Nursing and Midwifery Ethics. We were, at the time of the research, both staff nurses working in the intensive care field, Tom Last in North Wales and Nigel Self on the Isle of Wight. Of great assistance to the study were Paul Wainwright, then Professional Officer at The Welsh National Board for Nursing, Midwifery and Health Visiting, and Clive Harries, Research and Development Officer at Hinchingbrooke Hospital, Huntingdon. Some statistical analysis was undertaken by John Kassab, Head of Statistics at the University of Wales at Bangor. A preliminary and briefer version of our findings was published in the *British Journal of Nursing* (Last *et al.* (1992)).

Notes

1   Of course, this has the disadvantage that it is not based on a survey of what ICU nurses in general think. Furthermore, we are aware that we are perhaps leading the respondents by conceiving the question as one of 'extension'. For a list of other procedures which respondents themselves thought could legitimately be regarded as extending the nursing role, see Last *et al.* (1992).

References

Department of Health and Social Security (1977) *The extending role of the clinical nurse – legal implications and training requirements.* Joint Working Party, DHSS, London.

Jarvis A., Moores Y., Haughey A. & Bull M. (1992) *The extended role of the nurse/ Scope of professional practice.* PL/CNO(92)4 (England), CNO(92)9 (Wales), CNO(92)3 (Scotland), CNO(92)2 (N. Ireland). DoH, London.

Last T., Self N., Kassab J. & Rajan A. (1992) Extended role of the nurse in ICU. *British Journal of Nursing* **1**(13), 672–675.

Rowden R. (1987) The extended role of the nurse. *Nursing-Oxford* **3**(14), 516–517.

United Kingdom Central Council for Nursing, Midwifery and Health Visiting (1992) *The Scope of Professional Practice.* UKCC, London.

Welsh National Board (1990) *The Extended Role of The Nurse. A Discussion Paper.* Welsh National Board for Nursing Midwifery and Health Visiting, Cardiff.

Yellowkeys H. & Friend P. M. (1977) *The extending role of the clinical nurse – legal implications and training requirements.* Accompanying lettter CMO(77)10, CNO(77)9. Department of Health and Social Security, London.

Chapter 9
The Role of the Practice Nurse

Introduction

The extended or expanded role has been a vexed issue for many nurses working in the general practice setting, and may continue to be so. After the abolition of localised extended role certificates in line with the recent *The Scope of Professional Practice* document of the United Kingdom Central Council, it could become more difficult for practice nurses to say No to General Practitioners (GPs) who ask them to carry out tasks for which they have not been trained. Cook (1992b) suggests that GPs could also see this change as 'an opportunity to develop physicians' assistants', which would be cheaper.

There are other difficulties. Cook points out that, 'the rules relating to enrolled nurses in general practice at present are vague and lead to discrimination against them'. Practice nurse vulnerability also extends to their lack of a management structure, absence of support from a Health Authority and a limited availability of appropriately qualified practice nurse lecturers or assessors. Anxieties have been expressed by nurses in general practice regarding the funding of leave to meet the requirements expected in future for mandatory continuing education linked with re-registration.

In respect of their salaries, one of the initial problems for practice nurses is that there is no system to ensure that they are paid in a uniform way. 'In many FHSAs [Family Health Service Authorities arbitrary decisions are made on how the clinical gradings are applied', comments Johns (1989).

Educational initiatives throughout the United Kingdom have developed randomly, with a requirement from some FHSAs for new employees to attend an induction course, and no requirements in others. In addition, a plethora of schemes exist, from courses enabling practice nurses to enhance their skills on a part-time basis, to modular university diplomas whose philosophy is founded on research-based practice in an environment of shared learning. The venue, mode of delivery and the time of day of courses frequently make it difficult for a practice nurse to obtain release from her place of employment.

Historical background

Nurses have worked in the general practice setting since 1911 (RCN 1991). Often their nursing role was secondary to that of a receptionist, where answering the telephone and responding to the general practitioner's administrative requests in a quiet, predictable setting was their prime responsibility. When advertised, this part-time post could be found in small print in a local paper. Grateful for a position which fitted in with their domestic responsibilities the interviewee would rarely challenge the GP on the assurance of a job description, contract or National Insurance contributions. The possibility of job satisfaction was rarely considered. The GP rarely required the candidate to provide evidence of a professional qualification, references, a record of previous employment or appropriate continuing education. There was no formal educational preparation for the role.

In 1965, when GPs were first able to claim reimbursement for part of the salaries paid to practice nurses, it was estimated that there were 244 full-time practice nurses in England and Wales. By 1987 there were 6065, of which 96% worked part-time, equating to 3150 whole-time equivalent posts. Increasingly their contribution to the primary health care team was being acknowledged, as was the importance of their ability to provide quality clinical care within the general practice in the setting of the health centre or surgery (RCN 1991). They had also begun voicing anxieties regarding the extension of their role. As Jeffree (1990) commented, 'Nurses should not take on extended role activities without having received the appropriate education and training so to do and having been assessed as competent'.

The majority of nurses who are employed in general practice are registered general nurses who may also have a district nursing or health visiting qualification or one or more of a variety of post-basic qualifications. In addition, a number of nurses other than those holding a general nurse qualification are employed as practice nurses. They include registered sick children's nurses, registered mental illness nurses, registered nurses for mental handicap, enrolled nurses (general), district enrolled nurses, and midwives. A considerable proportion of practice nurses have been in their post in excess of 14 years (Damant 1990). The role of some practice nurses includes other responsibilities such as practice management or reception (Welsh Office 1992).

The heterogeneity of the developing content and pattern of work of practice nurses has been described by Damant (1990) who also defined a range of social, professional, epidemiological and organisational variables as factors which contributed to the wide variations observed in their practice.

A recent definition hardly describes the complexity of the role which, it may be observed, has developed through economic expediency and not from a professional regulatory framework:

'A practice nurse should hold an appropriate qualification which is registered or recorded on the ... Professional Register maintained by the United Kingdom Central Council for Nurses, Midwives and Health Visitors (UKCC). This will normally be Registered General Nurse. Where activities are undertaken for which a specific qualification is required, for instance health visiting, midwifery or district nursing, the person will be expected to hold the appropriate qualification of Registered Midwife or a recordable qualification in District Nursing. In addition the Registered Midwife must be a practising midwife as defined in the UKCC midwives' rules. When the practice nurse holds the qualification of Enrolled Nurse (General) only and is registered on Parts 2 or 7 of the UKCC Professional Register, then he or she may only undertake a limited range of duties, having due regard to the skills of Enrolled Nurses contained within the nurse training rules of the UKCC.' (DoH 1990b)

Towards the end of the 1980s it was widely considered that the NHS was in need of reform (Roberts 1992). The Government response was to introduce a policy based on 'less bureaucracy, less centralisation and less deference to professional expertise, more self-help, more conscious participation and more tolerance of diversities' (Klein 1989). A study by Enthoven in 1985 had suggested that GPs were hindering the reform of the National Health Service because they were politically powerful and had no desire to give up their autonomy. It was not surprising therefore, that general practice was the clinical discipline most affected by the Government's proposals, which included medical audit and increased accountability. The rationale behind this was that by changing the role of the 'gatekeeper to the NHS' (DOH 1989a) one could effectively alter the nature of the health service as a whole.

The autonomy and independence of GPs had been reinforced by the formation of the Royal College of General Practitioners (RCGP) in 1952 and the introduction of the Family Doctor's Charter in 1965. The RCGP had been formed to ensure that general practice was recognised as an important clinical discipline and was not seen, as it had been in the past, as peripheral to hospitals and consultants. The 'Family Doctor's Charter' was introduced to appease the profession, who maintained that the capitation system as the sole means of payment tended to result in a mediocre service from a large proportion of family doctors. Among its recommendations was an assurance that GPs would receive payments for preventative services, for employing a practice nurse and ancillary staff, and for limited educational opportunities.

In 1986 the Government issued proposals for the reform of primary health care in the form of a discussion document, 'Primary Health Care: An Agenda for Discussion' (DoH 1987b). Reiterating the themes suggested by the Griffiths Report (DoH 1978) it focused on the consumer-orientated and managerial aspects. Later the White Paper, 'Promoting Better Health' (DoH 1987a), based on the discussion document, remained faithful to the majority of its proposals. In addition, it emphasised a new governmental objective, that of 'the promotion of health and the prevention of disease', and called upon family doctors to initiate these changes in the form of screening, immunization and health promotion sessions. This was not an innovation for some practice nurses.

Further reforms with implications for general practice were identified in the White Paper, 'Working for Patients' (DoH 1989a), which pledged to 'extend patient choice, to delegate responsibility to where the services are provided and to secure the best value for money'. General practice was to be strengthened in four areas: patient choice; medical audit; prescribing costs; and management. Where 'Working for Patients' gave GPs increased work and responsibility in respect of the buying of hospital services for patients, the 1990 GP Contract (DoH 1989b) expanded their workload with an expectation of further provisions designed to benefit the patient as a consumer.

Among the services eligible for financial entitlements were minor surgery, reaching targets in immunisation and cytology, screening, child health surveillance and health promotion clinics. It was evident that GPs could not achieve these targets without an increase in professional support.

There was a clear warning to GPs within the GP Contract and the 'Red Book' *Statement of Fees and Allowances* (DoH 1990a), that in delegating treatments or procedures, they must be sure that the person to whom they delegated such a treatment or procedure was competent to carry it out. Within some Family Health Service Authorities there was a four-fold increase in the employment of practice nurses at that time. In addition to a discretionary funding of 70% of their salary, the GP could now receive direct reimbursement for staff training.

Stanley (1989) commented, 'I wholeheartedly support the emergence of practice nurses with a wide range of skills overlapping with and complementary to those of GPs'. He avoided being distracted by the notion that the skills required of this generalist nurse were best met by 'the extended role of the practice nurse' or a 'nurse practitioner'.

Perhaps as a result of the efficiency of practice nurses, a new system of payments for the hitherto financially remunerative Heath Promotion Clinics was announced by the Government in June 1992. In future the FHSA will be firmly involved in working with practices to set targets for health promotion. There will be three bands of payment as opposed to the open-ended nature of the remuneration which created disparities in income between practices.

Practice nurses were incensed, noted Cook (1992a), by the suggestion that 'there will be no more clinics' and adds, 'I have even heard that there will be no more practice nurses'. Mead (1992) maintains, however, that the practice nurse 'will still be one of the key players, with an extension of her current responsibilities to include a knowledge of audit and computer literacy'. Nevertheless as the growth in numbers of practice nurses arose out of a political whim in 1989, so their numbers could equally easily decrease with the introduction of a new system of health promotion payments in 1993.

Promoting better health

Promoting Better Health, which was released in November 1987 by the Department of Health emphasised a new objective of 'the promotion of health and the prevention of disease' and called upon family doctors to initiate these changes in the form of screening, immunization and health promotion sessions.

The document makes evident the Government's belief that the service offered by general practice needed strengthening in four areas: patient choice; medical audit; prescribing costs; and management. Accordingly the changes for general practice implied by the White Paper were:

(1) the introduction of financial budgets including indicative pre-scribing budget and practice budgets;
(2) changes in GP's remuneration system, including an amendment of *The Statement of Fees and Allowances* (the 'Red Book') and a payment for minor surgery carried out in the practice (DoH 1990a);
(3) more choice for patients, for example, enabling them to charge the GPs more easily, the advertising of GP services to attract custom, consumer surveys; and

(4) greater emphasis on management with regards to FPC/FHSA composition and the number of GPs in practice.

Practice budgets were a fundamental proposal in 'Working for Patients', giving GPs in practices with over 9000 patients the chance to become a fund-holding practice. An increased emphasis on management was also a provision, the Government undertaking to control the number of GPs practising and to reduce their retirement age from 70. Additionally, and persisting with the theme of quantitative assessment, it announced plans to change the composition of FHSAs. Indeed a change in the name, from Family Practitioner Committee to Family Health Services Authority, was indicative of their new role and function.

Expanding on the notion of increased patient choice, the 1990 GP Contract made the following recommendations to improve the general medical service:

- giving patients better choice
- making the terms of service more specific
- amending the statement of fees and allowances
- strengthening the GPs' link with the FHSA
- ensuring greater value for money (DoH 1989b).

The Government stated two important aims in changing the GPs' terms of service: (1) to specify more clearly the service they are expected to provide; (2) to better inform FHSAs to enable them to monitor the quality of services. The terms of service also state that: professional health care staff are properly trained and qualified; the training allowance will be replaced by a postgraduate education allowance (to encourage continuing education); there will also be payments for minor surgery, for reaching targets in immunization and screening, child health surveillance, and health promotion clinics.

Ensuring greater value for money meant assessing practice teams, premises, information technology, prescribing, hospital referral and medical manpower. Consequently, it was decided that the FHSA would continue to meet 70% of the costs of practice staff (including training). It was becoming evident that the GP would require additional professional support in meeting the financially attractive requirements of the legislation, particularly in respect of:

- health promotion targets
- new registration checks
- annual visits to every patient on the list over 75
- increasing immunization and cervical cytology uptake

- minor surgery
- child health surveillance.

As a result of these contractual arrangements, it was estimated that by March 1992 the number of full-time equivalent practice nurses employed in England and Wales was approximately 13 500, a four-fold increase since 1987.

In the free market GPs should be involved in the commissioning process, as District Hospital Services contracts reflect GP referrals. There could be implications for nurses employed by a fund-holding practice in the new-style NHS, as these practices have the opportunity of moving their funds around under the three main budgets of prescribing, effective surgery and staff costs.

The implementation of 'Caring for People' (DoH 1989c) has been slowed down, being effected in 1993. The implementation of these reforms will involve a change in the evolving relationship which has been developed by the practice nurse and other members of the Primary Health Care team as they assume 'key' case-holding responsibilities.

The fundamental principles expressed in the *Children Act 1989*, which came into force in 1991, include the child's welfare, parental responsibility and ethnic issues. It is likely that in addition to patients approaching practice nurses for practical advice on issues affecting the welfare of their children they could have an increased role in the protection of children as a result of this new legislation.

Socio-economic influences

The practice nurse today works in a society with a growing demand for health care, partly because of technical advances and partly because of increased life expectancy (Seedhouse & Cribb 1989). In addition, the pressure on community services has increased and because of factors such as the isolation of urban life and the acceptance of the right to welfare support, more demand is being made upon the services offered by GPs. The knowledge and expertise of the population in relation to rights and expectancies is increasing, and the current climate of increased openness is reflected in laws enabling access to health and medical reports. This has encouraged more patients to take part in making decisions that affect their health care and has required a demystification of knowledge. The media, no doubt, has been powerful in supporting this trend. It is possible, suggest Seedhouse and Cribb (1989):

'to identify two major trends in health care. One trend has arisen from the initiatives of nurses working directly with people in need, the other has been generated from outside the health care system by people whose priorities are not necessarily derived from the principles of health care. The first trend is a move away from a purely medical model towards a more egalitarian, more participative and broader conception of health. This approach is not only concerned with disease treatment and cure, but with ensuring that the whole process of care is as active and enabling as possible. The second trend exists because external forces have sought to regulate the quantity of care available, seeking to limit spending. One consequence of this trend is that there are fewer resources available to many practitioners in health care.'

There is also an increasing value being given to *health*. Several decades ago the World Health Organization defined health as a 'state of complete physical, mental and social well-being, rather than solely as an absence of disease' (WHO 1976). This statement has its critics, who suggest that it omits to address the dynamic aspects of health. Perhaps the idea that health means having the ability to adapt continually to constantly changing demands, expectations and stimuli, is seen to be more acceptable (Ewles & Simnett 1985).

Nurses working in the community have often concentrated on preventative medicine and health education, recording health information and teaching health skills (RCN 1991) but such activities are likely to be limited in their effectiveness unless the local range of health promotion action is recognised and actively supported. 'Health Promotion is the process of enabling people to increase control over, and to improve, their health' (WHO 1984).

Smail (1990) suggests that:

'The roots of the health promotion movement lie in an appreciation of the fundamental determinants of health. It must be seen as a multisectional activity, involving the organisation of public health policies, community action, the creation of supportive environments and the developments of personal skill for health.'

In 1978 the World Health Organization's International Conference in Primary Care at Alma Ata suggested the following declaration:

'A main social target of governments, international organisations and the whole world community in the coming decades should be attainment by all peoples by the year 2000, of a level of health that will permit them to lead a socially and economically productive life – primary health care is the key to attaining this target' (WHO 1978).

The following definition of a Primary Health Care Team was adopted in 1978:

'A Primary Health Care Team is an independent group of general medical practitioners and secretaries and/or receptionists, health visitors, district nurses and midwives who share a common purpose and responsibility each member clearly understanding his or her own function and those of other members, so that they all pool skills and knowledge to provide an effective Primary Health Care service' (DoH 1978).

It is worth noting that the practice nurse is not mentioned in this statement.

A Primary Health Care Team today, however, in addition to practice nurses, could include the practice managers, community mental handicap and mental health nurses, social workers, therapists, dietitians, counsellors, dispensers and consumer group representatives. Their expertise would enhance the quality of care offered to a community.

The World Health Organization has suggested that:

'Health systems based on the primary health care approach, require personnel who have been trained to handle competently a number of responsibilities mainly concerning the community; promoting self-reliance in health care among families and individuals; collaborating with development sectors other than the health sector in promoting health and prevention of disease and disability; and extending health care coverage to all segments of the population. These roles and functions demand new forms and patterns of practice incorporating epidemiological, biostatistical, psychological, cultural, political and socio-economic elements, as well as a good knowledge of modern communication techniques and educational technology. Above all, they demand new attitudes and orientation' (WHO 1991).

This view has been reinforced in a number of key government documents, including 'The Health of the Nation' (DoH 1992) and 'The Strategic Intent and Direction for the NHS in Wales' (Welsh Office 1992).

Much criticism has been levelled regarding the viability of the concept of the Primary Health Care Team. Bowling (1981) defined the function of a team as 'the transfer of a task to a person of lower rank'. She suggested that the reluctance of GPs to consider change was related to an insecurity about their professional status and second rate image, compared with hospital medicine. One might think problems arise in teamwork because nurses do not view their relationship with doctors as that of colleagues. Campbell *et al.* (1987) comment that while physicians encourage a form of teamwork in which nurses are subordinate, nurses do seek mutual collegiality with physicians.

There is anecdotal and published evidence that some members of the Primary Health Care Team adopt self-isolating attitudes (Damant 1990). This was reinforced by the UKCC (1990) who claimed that 'for practice nurses the risk of professional isolation is greater than is the case for other nursing staff working with organisations and with professional colleagues'.

There is a need to ensure that an open and effective communication system prevails, despite the different conditions of employment, physical environments, the arbitrary divisions of labour and professional prejudices.

Professional influences

It has been suggested that the following are features of a profession, and they may be considered in relation to the role of the practice nurse:

- possession of a body of knowledge
- service to clients
- standard of practice
- ethical code
- accountability
- status.

Akinsanya (1990) maintains that the relationship between medicine and nursing is often based on the fact that nursing is heavily dependent on medicine for the knowledge that underpins its practice. Indeed Bendall (1977) noted that 'nursing has virtually no power, no status or role outside medicine'. This was reaffirmed by Damant (1990) who reported that some practice nurses identified task-orientated modes of practice which had a greater allegiance to medicine than to nursing or the primary health care team as a whole. It is debatable whether the body of knowledge which underpins the practice of nurses who are presently employed in general practice has prepared them for the diversities of the role.

The United Kingdom Central Council for Nursing, Midwifery and Health Visiting regulates professional education and in collaboration with the four National Boards determines the standard, kind and content of the proposed curriculum. This ensures that the public is looked after by safe practitioners, but their skills may be specific to their original registerable qualifications and not to the demands of a role which has been determined by the financial incentives of medical legislation.

It is also disputable whether the traditional nurse education would have prepared them for the diversity of the practice nurse role. Cook (1992a), for example, describes a range of activities including 'well man, well woman, well adolescent, winter well, well elderly, disease management, not forgetting stop smoking clinics, alcohol control clinics and diet and weight control clinics'.

One of the problems with basic nurse education in the past was its over-dependence on the nurse in training as essential manpower for the NHS. Traditional nurse education emphasised the giving of information and instruction in the learning of practical psychomotor skills, training for obedience, conformity and discipline. The role of the nurse in health promotion in particular may have been hindered by adherence to the traditional method of training:

> 'Our basic training does little to foster the understanding and skills needed to enable us to help people accept responsibility for their own health and illness. We receive little or no training in how to communicate effectively as health educators. Our education concentrates solely on the problem of disease and we do little to strive towards physical, mental and social well being. Our curriculum is deficient in the recognition of the wider areas of life which affect health and the health care provision' (Alderton 1983).

In future, nurses who successfully complete the curriculum described in Project 2000 (UKCC 1986) will have: an understanding of the individual in social context; a problem-solving approach to the delivery of care; a health rather than illness perspective; and an orientation towards an active role for the nurse in the hospital and community settings.

In order to prepare an educational pathway to enable future nurses to work in the traditionally identified roles within the community, the profession was asked to respond to the 'Proposal for the Future of Community Education and Practice' (UKCC 1991), a proposal which developed from work done as part of the 'Post-Registration Education and Practice Project' (PREPP) (UKCC 1990). Currently practising first level practice nurses were not among the group who would be automatically recognised, within the terms of these proposals, as community health care nurses and they were understandably aggrieved. However, the Registrar and Chief Executive Office of the UKCC (Ralph

1992) did say, 'I feel sure that pathways will be made available to practice nurses'. Practice nurses are hopeful that this will give recognition to their described area of specialist practice or body of knowledge. This will complement a course of educational preparation which should be shared wherever possible with other community health care nurses.

The education pathway for nurses currently working in general practice has developed in a haphazard manner. Influential representatives of the Royal College of General Practitioners with a keen interest in the training of practice nurses were members of the steering group who met to address this issue in 1980. In 1985 an outline curriculum which described a course of no less than 10 days and recommended for first level nurses only was published by the National Boards. The course was based on three areas of study: (1) professional development; (2) procedures and techniques to be used in the treatment room/health centre; and (3) management of the treatment room/health centre.

Although the regulations suggested that wherever possible the courses would be held alongside district nursing and health visitor courses, to encourage elements of shared learning, in practice they rarely met.

As their numbers increased, practice nurses were demanding a more comprehensive educational programme which reflected the Recordable or Registerable pathway available for other community nurses, despite the lack of funds which would enable them to study full time for an academic year. The English National Board's 'Review of Education and Training for Practice Nursing' (Damant 1990) recommended a course which would ensure a qualification recordable on the Professional Register of the UKCC.

This was somewhat in conflict with the ethos of continuing education frameworks which were being developed by the Welsh and Scottish National Boards for Nursing, Midwifery and Health Visiting. The current trend was for a common core course for practitioners from a variety of settings with the opportunity to enrol on further modules which the practitioners identified as pertinent to their role. This did 'free up' the body of knowledge, but practice nurses were still anxious to enhance their practical skills as demanded by the GP.

Service to clients

Traditionally, the general practitioner largely determined the service the practice nurse offered to the practice population. However the 'doctor-nurse game' as described by Dachelet (1978), which reinforced the view that nurses accept that only a physician can diagnose a health problem, is changing.

Practice nurses could present themselves as offering a service complementary *to* medicine rather than *for* medicine. They are in an ideal situation to support the Primary Health Care Team in the delivery of care, whose aims were described in 'Promoting Better Health' (DoH 1987a). The practice nurse is also in a key position to address what could be done to improve the service offered to clients as described in 'Nursing in the Community' (The Roy Report) (DoH 1990c). Three questions are asked: (1) What are the needs of the population served? (2) What skills are needed to fulfil those needs? (3) Who has acquired those skills through education and training?

Through close collaboration with other members of the Primary Health Care Team practice nurses have the experience to widen the availability of care to the patient population. Other members of the Primary health Care Team, however, became anxious regarding the widening availability of services offered by the practice nurse. Butterworth (1988) suggested that 'Promoting Better Health' had 'carved up some clearly held territory in health promotion and screening, offering it fair and square to family doctors and practice nurses'.

The UKCC responded with a 'Statement on Practice Nurses and Aspects of the New GP Contract' (UKCC 1990). This document noted the increase in the number of nursing staff directly employed by GPs and how this could affect the delivery of care offered by district nurses, health visitors and other nurses. The development of their nursing role in GP practices was seen to be acceptable, provided that any extension in their role was negotiated with them and was seen to build upon the core nursing role. To ensure the interest of the patient or client was best served, sound policies for practice were to be developed. GPs were to ensure that when they delegated treatment or procedures they 'must be satisfied that the person to whom they are delegating is competent to carry them out'.

Another feature of their service to clients has involved practice nurses in the production of the practice information leaflet which should be freely available and updated annually. Their responsibilities also extended to preparing the nursing contribution to the annual practice report which involves carrying out a quantitative audit of their work.

Standard of practice

The Royal College of Nursing (RCN) claims to represent 65% of all trained nurses. Similar to professional organisations in other occupational fields it has come to recognise that professional and labour relation issues are often inseparable. Standards of care, for example, depend heavily on adequate staffing levels and this has long been a subject of negotiation between management and union.

In the 1960s this commitment to quality assurance was formalised with the publication of the RCN's first 'Standards of Care Project' led by Baroness Jean MacFarlane. Since that time, a series of publications on guidelines for good practice or national standards for particular areas of nursing have been produced. A group representing practice nurses met regularly for 3 years to produce a document which was relevant to the role and to the right standards which are achievable, constructive and desirable. In placing the responsibility firmly on nurses to decide what constituted good nursing, practice and care, they reflected the aims of the Project. Achieving quality assurance in health care based on a patient-centred approach requires an understanding of the nursing philosophy, accountability, knowledge and skills and the appropriate management and educational programmes which support this aim.

The groups representing the Practice Nurse Forum of the RCN were encouraged to reflect upon their understanding of patient care and how it could be improved. It was essential that recognisable requirements for delivery of the service were identified and that they should be patient focused at all times, must be owned by clinical practitioners involved, must be multidisciplinary, and must be achievable.

Due to the complexities of the role their task in setting the standards was complex. Job descriptions, where they existed, were varied and this was compounded by differences in practice philosophies and the individual qualifications, experiences and competencies of practice nurses. It was therefore essential to address not only the standards for the practice nurse's work environment, but the job description and professional role within the primary health care team.

In 1989, comments on the first draft were invited from delegates at the Practice Nurse Conference and were incorporated into the final document. The broad areas of professional accountability, the work environment, health promotion, care in chronic disease, and acute care were incorporated into the final document (RCN 1991). In conclusion, Woodman comments that standard setting is only one part of the quality assurance cycle. Monitoring of the standard is essential. In addition, as one of the principles of standard-setting is ownership, the practice nurses would be encouraged to set standards for their own work within their own practice setting or group.

Once practice nurses are confident with their own standards, perhaps they should consider addressing one of the key recommendations for practice education and management made in a Queen's Nursing Institute

(1991) publication: 'The best model for quality assurance in primary care is a team working in concert to identify problems and improve care for families and communities'.

Accountability

Of particular concern to the practice nurse is clause four of the UKCC's *Code of Professional Conduct* which, in the second edition (1984), states: 'Acknowledge any limitations of competence and refuse in such cases to accept delegated functions without first having received instruction in regard to those functions and having been assessed as competent'. In the third edition (1992) the responsibility for competency is changed and the clause now reads: 'Acknowledge any limitations in your knowledge and competence and decline any duties or responsibilities unless able to perform them in a safe and skilled manner'.

Regarding the accountability of practice nurses, it has been suggested (RCN 1991) that practice nurses have no clearly defined professional or managerial structure behind them, which gives them a certain degree of autonomy. Johns (1989) however, suggests that in exercising this autonomy they are displaying a feature which is an important requisite of professional behaviour. The RCN addressed this issue in 1991, looking at the areas of:

(1) *Contract of employment and job description:* each practice nurse is expected to have a written contract of employment and job description.
(2) *Post-basic education:* each practice nurse is to attend an approved post-basic course prior to commencing work as a practice nurse or at least within the first year of practice.
(3) *Continuing education:* each practice nurse has the opportunity for regular updating and continuing education appropriate to her professional needs.
(4) *Communication within the Primary Health Care Team:* each practice nurse works in a collaborative and co-operative manner with health care colleagues.
(5) *Resources outside the Primary Health Care Team:* each practice nurse is responsible for knowledge of and access to resources for the benefit of the patient.
(6) *Developing written protocols:* each practice nurse develops protocols with appropriate members of the Primary Health Care Team.
(7) *Confidentiality:* as described in clause 9 of the Code of Conduct.

(8) *Management of time:* the practice nurse uses their skills and time effectively for the benefit of the patient.

Practice nurses, says Johns (1989), are well placed to forge working relations with doctor colleagues. Being held to account by doctors, he maintains, only presents attitudinal obstacles. Nevertheless the practice nurse, in being accountable directly to the GP without a nursing line of management, is without doubt vulnerable.

Status

For practice nurses, unlike district nurses or health visitors, there is no recordable or registratable post-basic qualification which prepares them for their role. In being employed by the GP, promotion through the traditional nursing pathway is not available for a practice nurse, neither is the support of a nursing line manager. Some FHSAs, however, are employing primary health care facilitators or nurse advisers who may advise GPs in the appointment of prospective staff, organise orientation and continuing education programmes and support practitioners. Their influence is variable.

Recent additions to the nursing journals available have included *Practice Nurse* and *Practice Nursing*, the publication of which could be associated with the manifestations of the GP Contract 1990. There has been a particular focus in *Practice Nurse* since 1989 on topics such as asthma, diabetes, family planning, health promotion, managing minor ailments, minor surgery, practical screening and women's health. These reflect areas which, if successfully introduced into the practice, would financially reward the GP.

Conclusion

To enable practice nurses to accommodate contemporary challenges and aspects of their expanding role the following need consideration:

(1) Opportunities for developments in UKCC rules to enable appropriately qualified practice nurses to obtain a Registered Nurse Teacher qualification.
(2) The development of a recognised practice teacher/mentor and route of preparation.
(3) Collaboration between the educational establishments and

National Boards regarding educational issues and uniformity of salaries.

(4) Opportunities for the appropriate second level nurses to convert to first level.

(5) Encourage FHSAs to appoint a bank of nurses to replace colleagues on study leave.

(6) Accommodate practice nurses who have district nursing or health visiting qualifications into 'Preparing for Prescribing' at a later date.

(7) Ensure that practice nurses have the educational preparation for audit and devising protocols.

(8) Appoint a nurse adviser/facilitator in each FHSA.

(9) Encourage collegiality between the Royal College of General Practitioners and the nursing bodies.

There are no doubt other important issues. All of them need to be addressed if we are to go beyond the situation described by Jane Salvage, a situation which still applies to practice nurses: 'part-time nurses, like other part-time women endure the usual disadvantages of low pay, job insecurity, lack of fringe benefits and poor promotion prospects' (Salvage 1985).

References

Akinsanya J. (1990) Reflections on being a professional. *Practice Nurse* **2**(8), 432–433.

Alderton J. S. (1983) In training, but I want to be educated. *Nurse Educatiton Today* **3**(2), 29–31.

Bendall E. (1977) The future of British nursing education. *Journal of Advanced Nursing* **2**, 171–181.

Bowling A. (1981) *Delegation in General Practice. A Study of Doctors and Nurses.* Tavistock Publications, London.

Butterworth C. A. (1988) *Breaking the boundaries: new endeavours in community nursing.* Inaugural lecture, University of Manchester.

Campbell A., Heider N. & Pollock T. (1987) Barriers to physician–nurse collegiality. An anthropological perspective. *Social Science and Medicine* **25**(5), 421–425.]

Cook R. (1992a) Dancing queen. *Practice Nursing*, March, 23.

Cook R. (1992b) Healthy new arrivals. *Practice Nursing*, July/August, 2.

Dachelet C. (1978) Nursing's bid for increased status. *Nursing Forum* **17**.

Damant (1990) *The Challenges of Primary Health Care in the 1990s. A Review of Education and Training for Practice Nursing. The Substantive Report.* ENB.

Department of Health (1978) *The Primary Health Care Team.* Standing Medical Advisory Committee (SMAC). DoH, London.

Department of Health (1987a) *Promoting Better Health,* Command No. 249. DoH, London.

Department of Health (1987b) *Primary Health Care: An Agenda for Discussion.* DoH, London.

Department of Health (1989a) *Working for Patients.* DoH, London.

Department of Health (1989b) *General Practice in The National Health Service: The 1990 Contract.* DoH, London.

Department of Health (1989c) *Caring for People: Community Care in the Next Decade and Beyond,* DoH, London.

Department of Health (1990a) *Statement of Fees and Allowances* (paras. 52, 53). DoH, London.

Department of Health (1990b) *A Definition of Practice Nurse.* DoH, London.

Department of Health (1990c) *Nursing in the Community* (Roy Report). DoH, London.

Department of Health (1992) *The Health of the Nation.* DoH, London.

Enthoven A. (1985) *Reflections on tthe Management of the NHS. The Nuffield Provincial Hospitals Trust.* Nuffield, London.

Ewles L. & Simnett I. (1985) *Promoting Better Health. A Practical Guide to Health Promotion.* Wiley, Chichester.

Jeffree P. (1990) Practice nurse training. *Practice Nurse* **3**(4), 145.

Johns C. (1989) Accountability and the practice nurse. *Practice Nurse* **2**(7), 303–334.

Klein R. (1989) *The Politics of the NHS.* Longman, London.

Mead M. (1992) Health promotion. Gazing into the crystal ball. *Practice Nurse* **5**(3), 173.

Queens Nursing Institute (1991) *Quality Through Teamwork.* QNI and NAQUA, London.

Ralph C. (1992) Comment. *Practice Nursing,* July/August, 2.

Roberts M. H. M. (1992) *GPs in the NHS: The Politics of Budgets and Etthics.* Unpublished Dissertation, Sussex University, Brighton.

Royal College of Nursing (1991) *Standards for Practice Nursing.* Scutari, London.

Salvage D. (1985) *The Politics of Nursing.* Heinemann, London.

Seedhouse D. & Cribb A. (1989) *Changing Ideas in the Health Service.* Wiley, Chichester.

Smail S. (1990) Health promotion and the new GP contract. *Practice Nurse* **5**(3), 173.

Stanley I. (1989) The nurse partner. *Practice Nurse* **1**(10), 432–433.

United Kingdom Central Council for Nursing, Midwifery and Health Visiting (1984) *Code of Professional Conduct for the Nurse, Midwife and Health Visitor,* 2nd edn. UKCC, London.

United Kingdom Central Council for Nursing, Midwifery and Health Visiting (1986) *Project 2000. A New Preparation for Practice.* UKCC, London.

United Kingdom Central Council for Nursing, Midwifery and Health Visiting (1990) *Report of the Post-Registration Education and Practice Project.* UKCC, London.

United Kingdom Central Council for Nursing, Midwifery and Health Visiting (1990) *Statement on Practice Nurses and Aspects of the GP Contract.* UKCC, London.

United Kingdom Central Council for Nursing, Midwifery and Health Visiting (1991) *Report on the Proposals for the Future of Community Education and Practice.* UKCC, London.

Welsh Office (1990) *Strategic Intent and Direction for the NHS in Wales.* Welsh Office, Cardiff.

Welsh Office (1992) *Practice Nursing.* Welsh Nursing and Midwifery Committee, Welsh Office, Cardiff.

World Health Organization (1976) *Basic Documents.* WHO, Geneva.

World Health Organization (1978) *Report on Intended Conference on Primary Health Care* (Alma Ata, USSR). WHO, Geneva.

World Health Organization (1984) *Education and Training of Nurse Teachers and Managers with Special Regard to Primary Health Care.* WHO, Geneva.

World Health Organization (1991) *Nursing in the Primary Health Care. Ten Years After Alma Ata and Perspectives for the Future.* WHO, Geneva.

Chapter 10
The Enhanced Role of the Midwife

Introduction

This chapter will look at how in certain areas within the United Kingdom and abroad the role of the midwife has been exercised and enhanced. It is interesting to see the efforts that are being made by midwives, in the face of political and/or medical opposition, to retain and regain their role and resist attempts by management forces to specialise within their sphere of practice and to lose their holistic pattern of care. Also the educational opportunities required to facilitate midwives fulfilling their role will be considered: these include pre-registration midwifery education and programmes developed to enhance and maximise the role of the clinical midwife.

Definitions and prohibitions

The role of the midwife as laid down by the International Confederation of Midwives/International Federation of Gynaecologists and Obstetricians and supported by the World Health Organization is as follows:

'A midwife is a person who, having been regularly admitted to a midwifery educational programme, duly recognised in the country in which it is located, has successfully completed the prescribed course of studies in midwifery and has acquired the requisite qualifications to be registered and/or legally entitled to practise midwifery.

She must be able to give the necessary supervision, care and advice to women during pregnancy, labour and the postpartum period, to conduct deliveries on her own responsibility and to care for the newborn and the infant. This care includes preventative measures, the detection of abnormal conditions in mother and child, the procurement of medical assistance and the execution of emergency measures in the absence of medical help. She has an important task in health counselling and education, not only for the women, but also within the family and the community. The work should involve antenatal education and preparation for parenthood and extends to certain areas of gynaecology, family planning and child care. She may practise in hospitals, clinics, health units, domiciliary conditions or in any other service.' (International Confederation of Midwives/International Federation of Gynaecologists and Obstetricians 1992)

Midwifery is unusual among the caring professions in that midwives are not involved solely or primarily in activities such as the prevention of illness (as with public health nurses), the treatment of individuals experiencing illness or the support of people with long-term health deficits. Midwifery, whilst encompassing a significant health education and promotion component, is concerned with the support of the childbearing woman and her family during *normal* physiological events. It is true, however, that the midwife in less developed countries may exercise a wider remit than in the West with a role as public health advisor for the woman and her family with a particular emphasis on child care, fertility and other women's issues (Royston & Armstrong 1989).

Where the scope of midwifery practice is under statutory control, the extent to which the midwife can fulfil the ICM/FIGO definition varies. Further restrictions can and often do occur due to local custom and practice. In the United Kingdom the midwife provides care and support to the mother and newborn for up to 28 days after birth, whereas in Italy the period of child surveillance lasts until the child is 3 years old (Oakley & Houd 1990). Visiting the pregnant woman or mother and her new baby at home occurs in Denmark, the Netherlands and the United Kingdom, while midwives in Germany, Italy and Greece have little if any involvement in antenatal care (WHO 1985). Nurse-midwives in the United States of America support the woman in between her pregnancies providing general health surveillance and gynaecological screening (Silverton 1988).

The midwife, as laid down in the ICM/FIGO definition, is the practitioner of the normal and, although part of her role is the definition of the abnormal, it is at this point that she may relinquish responsibility (albeit temporarily) for the planning and supervision of care. She may at that time follow medical orders while continuing to give care and emphasising those aspects of the childbearing process which remain normal (as is common in the United Kingdom), or she may, as can occur in the United States of America, be obliged to hand over care to medical and nursing colleagues.

DeVries (1989) argues that in the USA childbirth has passed from a state of scientific care with its readiness to intervene, to one of control and 'active passivity' which, whilst espousing non-intervention, is so controlling by its use of monitoring to ensure normality as to be almost constantly intervening. Indeed, such a rationale for care lies behind some limits which have been placed upon midwifery practice.

In California the state law which governs the practice of nurse-midwives, prohibits them from using any instrument to assist the birth of the child (with the exception of those to clamp and cut the umbilical cord) or from prescribing or administering before or during birth drugs or medications other than laxatives or disinfectants. Failure to summon the advice and assistance of a doctor for named conditions in pregnancy, labour and the puerperium can lead to the loss of the midwife's practice licence (DeVries 1989). Even in the case of licensed midwives (non-nurses who have undergone either an apprenticeship and/or a classroom-based programme) their practice can be severely prescribed. Licensed midwives in Arizona are expressly forbidden from attending any woman aged 35 years or over irrespective of previous history or presence of risk factors (DeVries 1989).

It has been shown that women over the age of 35 years do not form a uniformly high-risk group; for those who are healthy and of good socioeconomic status there is little risk (Silverton 1993).

Midwifery practice is by its very definition holistic in nature, concerning itself with the whole process of childbearing from preconception care to breast-feeding advice and with the woman as a part of her family and immediate social group. It also encompasses not simply the physical aspects of care but the engendering in the woman of a feeling of spiritual wellbeing, empowerment and control over her own body (Oakley 1976; Oakley & Houd 1990); such a total approach needs to be learnt from the start of practitioner education.

Midwives in the United Kingdom can be the point of first contact with the health service for a pregnant woman, can give all antenatal care, undertake care and supervision in labour and during birth, and then care of the mother and newborn for a period of up to 28 days. During this time the woman need have no other contact with another health care worker, although in reality women can meet in excess of three dozen different people during this time (Flint 1991).

Historically medicine has sought through legislation to limit midwifery practice to that which supports and complements but does not compete with obstetrics (Arney 1982). The move in the focus of midwifery practice from the community into hospital, facilitated the imposition of protocols and policies which specify the boundaries of normality and of the practice of midwives within them (Tew 1990).

The increase in scientific knowledge about childbirth produced a change from the process being viewed as one of mystery, with midwives defining the boundary between normality and abnormality, to one where normality can only be diagnosed in retrospect following comparison of events with accepted guidelines. This has further circumscribed the practice of midwifery (Arney 1982; Oakley 1976, 1984). However, the legal basis of midwifery practice as laid down in the UK in the 'Midwives' Rules' (UKCC 1991) has always permitted and encouraged midwives to fulfil their role in the care and support of women having a normal pregnancy, birth and postnatal period and of the well newborn.

Enhancing the midwifery role

Prior to *The Scope of Professional Practice* (UKCC 1992) midwives in this country were to a large part exempt from the debate regarding the extended or expanded role of the nurse, which tended to revolve around specific skills and competencies rather than the totality of practice. This document has now defined what is and what is not meant by role expansion in a way which makes it much more relevant to midwifery.

For the most part midwives who are seeking to enhance their role are doing so in two main areas. The first of these is the recapturing of the full extent of the traditional midwives' role. The second is the acquisition of new skills to extend her involvement with the woman, such as those relating to health promotion and screening or to more technical interventions such as the use of vacuum extractors for birth, and the prescribing and administration of oxytocic drugs within agreed protocols. The certification of competence for an extended role has not been an issue in midwifery, although some UK obstetric units still require them before midwives can top up epidurals.

Midwives seeking to exercise their role to the full have often been constrained by the bureaucracy surrounding maternity care or by medical control to such an extent that some have gone into practice outside traditional structures (Oakley 1976; Oakley & Houd 1990). These alternative patterns of practice are not always sanctioned by health care organisers to whom independent practice and/or the supporting of women to give birth at home can be seen to undermine the dominant mode of operation. Where midwives have formed self-help groups they have found it hard for their voices to be heard.

The Association of Radical Midwives' blueprint for practice, *The Vision*, was launched in 1986 and whilst applauded by many midwives had only a limited impact on practice. Its recommendations for the full use of midwifery skills, continuity of care, choice in childbirth and accountability of the service to the women who use it were echoed in the

UK Government's Health Committee Report (Health Committee 1992). However, many of the Committee's findings were ignored by the Government, especially where they do not accord with current medical opinion (Department of Health 1992). An expert advisory committee was subsequently established by the Government to explore ways in which its response to the Health Committee Report could be implemented.

The Government's initial response was somewhat cautious and did not support many recommendations even where supported by research (Department of Health 1992). This was particularly evident in relation to birth at home, the provision of maternity services in small midwifery/family doctor units and the continued involvement of medical staff in the antenatal care of normal women (shared care). A cynical view could be taken that the midwife will only be 'allowed' to practise with an enhanced role either where the doctor wishes to relinquish an aspect of care or where a midwife is significantly cheaper to employ. In the latter case, however, were the midwife to be appropriately rewarded for the work she undertakes and the level of responsibility she assumes, the financial advantage would disappear.

This has occurred in New Zealand where midwives have reasserted themselves with the support of women's groups. Their practice was severely restricted by both the medical establishment and the nursing profession who controlled midwifery (Donley 1986). There had been no midwifery training in the country since 1979 and such midwifery practices as existed were totally under medical control; indeed, nurses could undertake obstetric care under medical supervision. Despite opposition from obstetricians and the national Nursing Council, midwifery practice and education have been recognised by an amendment to law (Stodart 1990). Midwives will no longer need to hold a nursing qualification and they will be employed as contracted care providers with a similar role in maternity care and fee structure as family doctors. It has been necessary to provide re-education and support for existing midwives who had not been permitted to practise and had lost confidence in their ability to fulfil their role (Donley 1990).

Choice and medical dominance

Dissatisfaction with the hospital-based and medically-led form of care has prompted some women to demand a different form of care, be it birth centres in the USA, or home birth and/or the services of an independent or team midwife in the UK (Oakley & Houd 1990). Lack of consultation regarding modes of care and use of inappropriate or non-valid technology (the value of which is not supported by research) had prompted some women choosing a hospital birth to produce plans for their care detailing what they would wish to happen.

Many midwives supported these women in their choice whilst others, adopting a medical-support role of 'obstetric nurse', resented their position as 'expert' being challenged. They had forgotten that 'midwife' means 'with woman', which implies a relationship of equality rather than one of unequal power. To a lesser degree the women's dissatisfaction has also manifested itself in the setting up of lay groups to address deficiencies in the service. These have included parent education and breast-feeding counsellors and support groups (DeVries 1989). It is indeed an indictment of the provision of such a central portion of midwifery care that some women, feeling their needs are unmet, have sought recourse to outside support.

The Health Committee Report (1992) on the maternity services indicated quite clearly that the service as currently provided for the majority of women was too medically based and did not meet their needs.

The midwives' role has grown gradually due to changes in the approach and management of care; these have not always been to the benefit of women and their families. Care needs to be taken that all such changes are to the benefit of the woman and her family and not simply due to managerial convenience.

The acknowledgement of the need to give total care has resulted in midwives undertaking repair of the perineum or requesting antenatal investigations. The move of place of birth from home to hospital (with its assumption of pathology) brought with it the application of regimes more suited to the care of the ill than well people (Arney 1982; Schwarz 1990). In addition, the prevailing obstetric culture of 'normality' being determined only in retrospect has resulted in midwives having to fight against the introduction of technology rather than wholeheartedly embracing it (as may be the case in acute nursing).

In the UK the reduction in the hours worked by junior hospital doctors has resulted in an examination of who should do what in the field of hospital-based health care. This has coincided with a reduction in hospital-based antenatal clinics and the realisation that some medical tasks were actually prompted by midwives. Foremost amongst these is the transfer home of a woman following normal birth, the responsibility for which used to lie with the junior doctor although it was the midwife who told him which women were fit to go home.

Midwives should resist the imposition of medical duties onto their role where this is simply due to the exigencies of the service. However, it could be argued that where it would permit the midwife to give total care to women (as with the assessment for transfer home) it should be adopted following suitable preparation.

Changes in the running of the health service in the UK (the estab-lishment of speciality-based directorates and the purchaser/provider split, for example) together with a scarcity of financial resources has made it all the more necessary that the role of the midwife is further examined.

Flint (1991) has shown how total care from a small group of midwives produces similar outcomes in terms of perinatal mortality and maternal morbidity (whilst significantly improving maternal satisfaction and reducing cost) as does obstetrician-led care for women at low risk of complications. In 1982 the Maternity Services Advisory Committee recommended that the services of the obstetrician should be con-centrated primarily on those women at significant risk of complications. However, there is still a prevalent culture that results in women at low risk of complications seeing an obstetrician on a regular basis and having her labour and birth indirectly supervised by obstetric staff.

It has been shown in the Netherlands that community-based mid-wifery care produces outcomes which are better than those for hospital care, as regards perinatal mortality. In addition, the midwives were accurate in predicting those women needing to be referred for hospital-based obstetric care (given by midwives under the direction of medical staff), this group experiencing the highest perinatal mortality rate (Van Alten *et al.* 1989).

Further force to the argument for the full use of midwifery skills came with the Health Committee Report (1992), which recommended mater-nal choice, consultation, continuity of care, a review of the routine use of technology and appropriate and full use of midwifery skills. Patterns for alternative modes of practice, such as group practices contracting to provide care within the NHS, independent practice and team midwifery, reflect a growing agreement within the profession that unless skills are used to the full they will disappear. A task-oriented approach will only hasten the employment of support workers to undertake what is part of the midwives' role (Clarke 1993).

Ultrasound

One specific area of practice which has resulted in expansion of the midwives' role is that of obstetric ultrasound. Such a role expansion is not without controversy. There have been arguments regarding the appropriateness of moving outside the accepted role definition (ICM/IFGO 1992) and diluting midwifery practice with the adoption of tech-nology which is still of incompletely proven value and safety for the woman at low risk of complications (Neilson & Grant 1989; Stewart 1986).

Furthermore, it is an encroachment into the role of another health professional – the radiographer. Whilst radiographers follow an 18-month intensive post-qualification diploma course, there is no such stipulation for doctors and midwives although there are voluntary programmes of shorter duration. It could also be argued that since, according to the 'Midwives' Rules' (UKCC 1991), on finding a deviation from the normal, the midwife is obliged to summon medical support, there is little advantage in using a midwife rather than a radiographer to perform this test. When midwives first started to perform obstetric ultrasound, radiographers were not permitted to give any feedback on the findings to mothers. Now that this situation has changed it could be argued that there is little place for midwives performing this test especially when they are prevented from exercising other more central aspects of their role.

The widespread use of midwives to perform ultrasound examinations could lead to more frequent use, which would not be in the mother's best interests (Taylor 1990). As has been argued with regard to intravenous cannulation, widely practised by American nurse-midwives, the possession of this skill has appeared to lead to a greater number of American women under midwifery care having an intravenous infusion sited 'just in case' than occurs in the UK where there needs to be a specific reason. Having the skill may make the practitioner more likely to perform the procedure (Silverton 1989).

Educational initiatives

The need to provide the British clinical midwife with skills and knowledge which she may not have acquired through her traditional programme of preparation has produced two different educational initiatives.

The first of these is the re-emergence of pre-registration midwifery programmes. The spur for these came as a result of a demographic reduction in the number of 18-year-olds projected to enter nurse training and a projected reduction in nurses available to train as midwives. A decision was made by the UK government to recruit older women, rather than school leavers, many of whom would have children of their own, a knowledge of the role of the midwife and a reluctance to undertake $4\frac{1}{2}$ years of preparation rather than 3 years to become a midwife.

As a result of economic circumstances, the expected reduction in recruitment to nursing did not occur but pre-registration midwifery diploma programmes have been available in the UK since 1990 and the numbers of courses are increasing. The entry into the profession of a significant number of midwives with no experience of nursing and its concomitant medical model of care should do much to promote midwifery autonomy, so long as clinical support staff act as role models for full midwifery practice.

Education to diploma level (which is now the only route into the profession for nurses as well as non-nurses) and above will also provide the practitioner with the skills and knowledge to argue for alternative modes of care and to question long-held beliefs. To this end clinical midwives are being actively encouraged to follow education programmes (to diploma and beyond) which have as their central element the improvement of clinical practice.

Such programmes provide the opportunity previously available to midwife teachers and managers to develop skills (both psycho-motor and cognitive) for professional development and improved client care. These programmes, many of which can be followed part-time (thus removing the need for managerial support and giving opportunities for part time staff), provide midwives with the means to question, to put together an argument, to highlight gaps in the research knowledge base and to advance the theoretical framework supporting practice.

Whilst educational opportunities have existed for midwives within the UK, for the most part these were theoretical in nature and entry to the courses was restricted by funding and service requirements. Programmes which practitioners can follow in their own workplace with flexible timing and costs will produce a wider dissemination of knowledge and skills. The skills as laid down for the schedule for enhanced midwifery practice take the competencies achieved at registration and develop them further rather than following a line of adopting medical duties. For example, the teaching of mothers and student midwives about the research basis to breast-feeding and the supporting of feeding mothers has been developed. The midwives' skills of assessment in pregnancy and labour take account not only of physiology but also of the psychosocial basis of care.

Conclusion

The situation regarding the scope of midwifery practice is one in which midwives are seeking to fulfil their role in the face of opposition from medical staff and health care providers. Midwives have to beware of taking on additional duties and expanding their role, especially where this is to suit managerial convenience rather than to meet the needs of mothers and babies.

Changes in the way in which midwives are prepared for their practice and further education for existing practitioners will support initiatives from inside and outside the profession for a fulfilment and enhancement of the midwives' role.

References

Arney W. R. (1982) *Power and the Profession of Obstetrics*. University of Chicago Press, Chicago.

Association of Radical Midwives (1986) *The Vision*. ARM, Ormskirk, Lancs.

Clarke R. (1993) The last stand? *Nursing Times* **89** (11), 36–37.

Department of Health (1992) *Maternity Services: Government Response to the Second Report from the Health Committee, Session 1991–92*. DoH, London.

DeVries R. G. (1989) Caregivers in pregnancy and childbirth. In *Effective Care in Pregnancy and Childbirth* (eds I. Chalmers, M. Enkin & M. J. N. C. Kierse), pp. 143–161. Oxford Medical, Oxford.

Donley J. (1986) An Interview. *Homebirth Australia* **9**, 6–7.

Donley J. (1990) Midwives' Dilemma. *Proceedings of the International Confederation of Midwives 22nd International Congress*, pp. 59–61. Midwives' Division of the Japanese Nurses' Association/Japanese Midwives' Association, Tokyo.

Flint C. (1991) The know your midwife scheme. In *Midwives, Research and Childbirth* (eds S.Robinson & A. M. Thomson), vol. 2, pp. 72–103. Chapman and Hall, London.

Health Committee (1992) *Second Report: Maternity Services*. Department of Health, London.

International Confederation of Midwives/International Federation of Gynaecologists and Obstetricians (1992) *Definition of the Role of the Midwife*. ICM, London.

Maternity Services Advisory Committee (1982) *Maternity Care in Action, Part I: Antenatal Care*. DoH, London.

Neilson J. & Grant A. (1989) Ultrasound in pregnancy. In *Effective Care in Pregnancy and Childbirth* (eds I. Chalmers, M. Enkin & M. J. N. C. Keirse), pp. 419–439. Oxford Medical, Oxford.

Oakley A. (1976) Wisewoman and medicine man: changes in the management of childbirth. In *The Rights and Wrongs of Women* (eds J. Mitchell & A. Oakley). Penguin, Harmondsworth.

Oakley A. (1984) *The Captured Womb*. Basil Blackwell, Oxford.

Oakley A. & Houd S. (1990) *Helpers in Childbirth: Midwifery Today*. Hemisphere, New York.

Royston E. & Armstrong S. (1989) *Preventing Maternal Deaths*. World Health Organization, Geneva.

Schwarz E. W. (1990) The engineering of childbirth: a new obstetric programme as reflected in British obstetric textbooks 1960–80. In *The Politics of Maternity Care: Services for Childbearing Women in Twentieth Century Britain* (eds G. Garcia, R. Kilpatrick & M. Richards), pp. 30–46. Clarendon Paperbacks, Oxford.

Silverton L. I. (1988) *Midwifery Education in the USA.* University College of Swansea, School of Social Studies, Swansea.

Silverton L. I. (1989) Letter. *Birth* **16**(1), 35.

Silverton L. I. (1993) The elderly primagravida. In *Midwifery Practice* (eds J. Alexander, V. Levy & S. Roch), vol. 4, pp. 74–90. Macmillan, London.

Stewart N. (1986) Women's views of ultrasonography in obstetrics. *Birth* **13**(1), 39–43.

Stodart K. (1990) After the Act. *New Zealand Nursing Journal* **83**(9), 21–22.

Taylor K. J. W. (1990) A prudent approach to ultrasonic imaging of the fetus and newborn. *Birth* **17**(4), 218–221.

Tew M. (1990) *Safer Childbirth? A Critical History of Maternity Care.* Chapman and Hall, London.

United Kingdom Central Council for Nursing, Midwifery & Health Visiting (1991) *Handbook of Midwives' Rules.* UKCC, London.

United Kingdom Central Council for Nursing, Midwifery and Health Visiting (1992) *The Scope of Professional Practice.* UKCC, London.

Van Alten D., Eskes M. & Treffers P. E. (1989) Midwifery in the Netherlands. The Wormerveer study; selection, mode of delivery, perinatal mortality and infant morbidity. *British Journal of Obstetrics and Gynaecology* **96**(6), 655–662.

World Health Organization (1985) *Having a Baby in Europe.* WHO, Copenhagen.

Chapter 11
Accident and Emergency and the Nurse Practitioner

Introduction

The publication of *The Scope of Professional Practice* (UKCC 1992b) brought to a close 15 years of frustration for accident and emergency nurses. This document emphasises the nurse's professional accountability and places decisions about the boundaries of practice in the hands of the individual practitioner. The Chief Nursing Officer at the Department of Health in England sees it as a major step forward and an opportunity for individual practitioners and their professional leaders and managers to build on past progress, examine practice afresh and further develop it in the interests of patient care (Moores 1992).

In June 1977 the health circular, 'The Extending Role of the Clinical Nurse: Legal Implications and Training Requirements', was published (DHSS 1977). This affected the role of the accident and emergency (A & E) nurse in a number of ways. Prior to 1977 many nurses were undertaking activities, for example the suturing of wounds, as a normal part of an experienced A & E nurse's role. Many experienced nurses were also assessing and treating patients with minor injuries and illnesses. This approach was an accepted part of A & E nursing, nurses extending their role through experience and teaching from more experienced colleagues. The sister in charge of the department would decide when nurses were able to extend their role and appropriate in-house training would be given.

One of the major problems with this method was the way nurses were taught new skills. The training was often inadequate, involving nothing more than observation, rather than being available as part of a structured development programme. After 1977 the situation with regard to the extension (or expansion) of the nurse's role in A & E became very muddled. Lists were drawn up of tasks normally carried out by the doctor but which could, with training, be undertaken by nurses. These tasks were often identified by health authority officers rather than by the nurses in the clinical area. Many tasks were removed from the nurse and this caused widespread frustration.

Another cause for concern was the way in which the extended role label was used to cover all nursing development. Jones (1986) found that restricted nursing practice in A & E, coupled with insufficient and inadequate post-basic education, resulted in deficiencies in the service. A survey of 411 nurses in 175 A & E departments covering 139 health authorities produced lists of procedures or tasks that health authorities had labelled 'extended'. The tasks ranged from application of plaster of Paris to crisis counselling, and from ear syringing to surgical procedures such as incision and drainage of small abscesses.

The most common extended procedures performed by nurses were stomach lavage (89% of respondents), suturing (50%), recording of ECGs (49%), administration of intravenous drugs (21%), venepuncture (13%), defibrillation (9%), intubation (9%), and IV cannulation and fluid replacement (4%). When asked about other duties, 64% of nurses said they were carrying out receptionist duties, 51% were providing domestic duties, and 77% were providing orderly work. Jones also found that an increase in direct nursing intervention could reduce patient waiting times by an average of 30 minutes, with savings of as much as 54 minutes in some cases.

The development of the ambulance paramedic in the 1980s did little to help nurses in A & E, who were by this time extremely frustrated with their restricted role. The vast majority considered the ambulance personnel to be less able than themselves yet they were being allowed to perform advanced life-support procedures, while the majority of nurses were being stopped. This frustration generated a great deal of animosity between the two groups of staff. It also highlighted the deficiencies of some A & E units in their response to the seriously ill or injured patient. Ambulance personnel, who now had a much higher knowledge base, and were able to perform advanced life-support, started to question the sometimes inadequate response of the nursing and medical staff who received the patient.

Cliff (1982) suggested that the role of the clinical nurse in A & E had not progressed as rapidly as that of the medical staff in A & E medicine. He also argued that A & E care should develop as a team concept and that the nurses must be part of that team. Walsh (1985b) considered the phrase 'the extended role of the nurse' to be singularly irrelevant in the A & E setting. In 1986 the UKCC (Cole 1986) emphasised that they saw specialised roles not as an optional extra but as an integral part of a practitioner-centred division of labour, while Eaves (1987) suggested that A & E nurses ought to be campaigning for further education and involvement in the psychological and social sphere, while at the same time arguing for the adequate provision of experienced medical staff in accident units.

Salvage (1986) considered that if extending the nurse's role is necessary to serve a client or client group this should be supported. Jones (1984), following the judgement made by Mr Justice Popplewell in the case of Derek Owen, argued that if nurses were merely servants who obey commands from either doctors or health authorities, there is little point in having a code of conduct.

Moores (1992) identified two major problems with the guidance on the extended role of the nurse. The first was the waste of valuable training resources which was caused by the retraining of staff because neither previous training nor certificates from other authorities were recognised between employing authorities. Second and more importantly, the system of extended roles promoted a task-based approach to care delivery and militated against comprehensive team-based holistic care.

As the 1980s progressed A & E nurses were gradually developing their role. Wright (1986) described the development of nursing support roles for the bereaved and for staff in crisis. Wright suggests that people in the front line of health care are often ill-equipped to deal with crisis or psychiatric emergency, pointing out that, 'It seems incredible that we are equipped for the most serious medical emergency but not for the crisis that may accompany it'. Blythin (1988) and Jones (1988) were pushing forward the development of triage. Blythin argued that traditional methods of patient reception do little to deal with the problems of overcrowding, missed diagnosis, inappropriate attenders or the provision of a quality service. Triage seeks to challenge many of these problems.

In 1986 the first nurse practitioner scheme was introduced at Oldchurch Hospital in Romford. Although this concept was not new in respect of small GP-run departments, this was the first time it had been attempted in a major department. The purpose of the scheme was to provide patients with a safe nursing opinion, to assess each patient's problem and request the necessary treatment, to record accurately each patient's problem and to maintain good communications within the department concerning patients. The scheme proved successful and has been introduced into a number of departments throughout the UK.

A & E nursing: a developing speciality

Two reports from the National Audit Office (NAO) indicate that A & E attendances continue to rise (NAO 1992a, 1992b). In 1990–1991, 11.2 million new attenders were seen in England and 1.2 million in Scotland. In both reports the NAO recommend a review of how A & E departments can make better and wider use of nurses' skills. Examples given are the development of triage to assess patients' needs and the extension of nurses' roles.

The NHS Management Executive (NHSME) have, in response to the reduction in junior doctors' working hours, produced a guidance document on making the best use of the skills of nurses and midwives (NHS Management Executive 1992). The NHSME recognise that attempting to create a list of procedures which might appropriately be performed by nurses would militate against the development of working practices which are appropriate in some local circumstances but not in others. Instead, plans for sharing care in a particular setting and speciality should be agreed by the medical and nursing professions locally.

The Scope of Professional Practice, although produced after this statement, supports this view. *The Scope of Professional Practice* indicates that the change in the development of professional practice must be based on principles which should govern adjustments to the scope of professional practice. This change has consequences for managers of clinical practice and professional leaders of nursing who must ensure that local policies and procedures are based on principles set out in the paper and in the Council's code of professional conduct. Any local arrangements must ensure that registered nurses are assisted to undertake, and are enabled to fulfil any suitable adjustments to their scope of practice.

Ashcroft (1992) considers that many tasks undertaken by doctors could be performed by nurses, and they should not wait until told to take on a new task, but should actively seek to gain experience. This change would also be in the best interests of the patient.

The Patients' Charter (Department of Health 1992) has major implications for nursing in the A & E department. Seven out of the nine national charter standards could have been written specifically for A & E departments. Charter standard 5 (waiting time for initial assessment) and charter standard 6 (respect for privacy, dignity and religious and cultural beliefs), for example, are embodied in the development of bereavement and crisis support being undertaken in many departments.

The way forward

A Strategy for Nursing (Department of Health 1989) identifies nursing as responding to human needs. Jones (1990) points out that in the A & E setting, all manner of human needs exist, and the philosophy of any A & E department must take this into account. Care should be based on a model of nursing, triage, and a problem-oriented approach encompassing assessment, problem identification, goals, intervention and evaluation (Fig. 1 in Appendix IV). All care should be documented.

To achieve these aims A & E nurses need a development programme which takes the nurse from orientation to the speciality through to becoming an advanced practitioner. Such a programme should provide a continuum from novice to advanced practitioner. The following sections of this chapter will describe such a programme in some detail (Fig. 2 in Appendix IV).

Development programmes for A & E staff should be developed locally but should include nationally recognised key subjects which would allow the nurse to move between departments without the need to start the programme again. It should also include some of the already available nationally recognised courses such as those approved by the National Boards. Through the integration of national courses and key subject material into a locally based development framework the professional development of the A & E nurse will provide both national standards of A & E nursing care and the best care for the local community.

The expanding role of the nurse should be seen as a continuous process and not simply as allowing nurses to perform additional tasks which may or may not have once been the sole remit of the doctor. The nurse should no longer expect to be taught a particular skill, unless it is part of the total development programme. Suturing, for example, should not be taught except in the context of total wound management. Intubation should be taught as part of the total management of airways. Neither should be taught unless there is a need for the nurse to practise such activities, and it must always be to the better service of the client.

The development programme

A development programme should be based on a philosophy which allows all the staff to work to the same beliefs and goals.

The philosophy

Nursing in A & E must be based on assisting the individual to improve health and maintain quality of life. Patients have a right to independence and dignity. Patients have the right to understand their treatment and care and they must have their freedom of choice and wishes taken into account. Nursing care should be provided by skilled nursing staff who through a process of role expansion can respond to the individual needs of the patient. These needs will span the entire spectrum of the human condition, physical, social, and psychological.

From novice to clinical specialist

The nurse entering the speciality of A & E nursing comes with a knowledge base developed over three years of general training, plus any additional knowledge and skills acquired from experience in another speciality. The development programme to be described here is based on four levels of competency. Each level provides the nurse with the knowledge and skills required to practise at that level. The development programme takes account of the individual's knowledge and skill and allows for flexibility.

Each nurse identifies their individual needs from the four levels of the programme. An individual programme based on the nurse's needs will then be developed using levels one to four. Each nurse will start at level one but parts of each level may be by-passed if the nurse has already gained that knowledge and skill elsewhere. Thus, for example, a nurse who has worked in a coronary care unit would need to be taught how to assess a patient arriving with a complaint of chest pain, but would not at level one need to be taught how to nurse the cardiac patient or how to record an ECG. The same system of exemption would apply at level two if the nurse was already competent in the procedure of defibrillation.

The development programme can be linked to clinical grading and used as a marker for regrading staff. Used in conjunction with clinical grading the programme allows the nurse to decide what level of competency to develop and at what speed to progress. This approach allows nurses who may find the speciality difficult not to be pressurised into taking on activities that they feel unable to handle with confidence. A change of job description and title also helps distinguish the level of competency between nurses, and when included as part of the development programme provides a clear career structure within the speciality. Departments that work on a four grade clinical career structure, D, E, F, G, can link each level to a grade. Those who work on a three grade clinical career structure (D, E, G) can combine level three and level four into one level.

The nurse should include the stages of the development programme within their own personal profile and should also use the development programme as a means of fulfilling the post-registration requirements of the UKCC (Post-Registration Education and Practice Project, PREPP).

Level One

Level one (Fig. 3 in Appendix IV) is designed to prepare the new nurse in

A & E with the basic knowledge and skills necessary to provide safe practice while at the same time having the support of more senior staff. At this level the nurse should be able to undertake patient assessment, intervention, and evaluation based on a model of nursing.

Level Two

This level (Fig. 4 in Appendix IV) prepares the nurse to practise within the department without supervision. The nurse having completed level 2 should be able to perform triage, supervise a clinical area, act as a mentor or preceptor to qualified nurses and students, teach other nurses within the department, provide health education to members of the public and perform advanced life support when dealing with any patient who has need of such care. The nurse will become the named nurse for an individual or group of patients.

Level Three

This level (Fig. 5 in Appendix IV) is designed to prepare the nurse for a clinical management role, and to provide additional assessment and diagnostic skills, thus allowing the nurse to treat certain patients without reference to a doctor (the emergency nurse practitioner). The nurse will become the named nurse for an individual or a group of patients.

Level Four

This level (Fig. 6 in Appendix IV) is designed to prepare the individual to practise competently as a clinical nurse specialist in accident and emergency (advanced practitioner). Specific courses, lectures and workshops allow the nurse to develop an increased knowledge base in one or more specific areas of A & E nursing. The nurse will become the named nurse for an individual or a group of patients.

Management

Beyond the clinical development programme there should be a management programme which provides the nurse with the necessary training to competently manage the A & E department in today's NHS. The prime objective must be to have the A & E department as an independent unit (clinical directorate, care group, etc.) and for that unit to be managed by the A & E nurse either as a director of services or as an equal partner in the management team.

National Courses

The four National Boards for Nursing, Midwifery and Health Visiting validate a variety of courses of relevance to the A & E practitioner. The English National Board 'Course 199' can be taken either as part of the ENB 'Critical Care Course' or as a stand-alone course, although demand is in excess of places available. A short ENB 'Course 3' is available for A & E nurses who have been working in the A & E department for some time. Other Boards offer different structures, as for example the Welsh National Board's Framework for Continuing Professional Education. In this scheme a variety of modules are offered, many of which would be suitable for A & E nurses.

A recent exciting development in A & E education has been launched at Salford University in conjunction with Hope and Bolton School of Nursing. A critical care programme has been designed which incorporates a clinical teaching and assessing module, a diploma and a degree.

The content of the development programme

The model of nursing

A model of nursing is simply a framework that provides a structure to nursing care. It should be introduced early in the level 1 stage of the development programme. Nursing in the A & E department must be based on well established theoretical foundations. The model is the key to nursing within the department. Not only can direct patient care be designed around the model, the model provides an excellent tool in which to develop the education of the nurse in all aspects of A & E patient care.

Walsh (1985b) has argued that vague notions about helping people get better, or assisting the doctor are not adequate foundations for nursing. Jones (1990) suggests that any nursing model used in the A & E department must be able to integrate with the medical model in the same way that nurses and doctors integrate in the team approach to patient care. He visualises the nursing model encompassing the core of the medical model.

It is suggested that no one model of nursing is right for A & E. The use of many different nursing models are seen in the A & E setting. Many are adaptations of well known models and some are home grown. Walsh (1985b) favours Orem's model, while Jones (1990) recommends the Components of Life model. This model represents current practice and also takes account of more than one model of nursing, yet is a model in its own right.

The model is based around the belief that humans are individuals with individual human needs and that during their lifespan the individual is engaged with various self-care activities in an attempt to retain independence. Seven components of life comprising physical, human behavioural and social aspects can be identified and these must be kept in balance to maintain health and quality of life. Due to an event (physical or mental injury or illness) in the course of the individual's lifespan the balance between the various components can become upset and the ability to maintain health and quality of life will be disrupted. The individual identifies the A & E staff as the resource to assist them in the re-balance of the components, re-establishment of independence, and thus a continuation of physical, emotional and social comfort.

The documentation linked with the model should be introduced at an early stage in the nurse's orientation to A & E, but the emphasis must be that the model is about the way the nurse thinks and works.

Interpersonal skills (including bereavement support and care in crisis)

The A & E department is the window of the hospital and for many people it is the only contact they will have with the NHS. One of the components of life identified in the model of nursing recommended for use in A & E by Jones (1990) is 'communication'. This component is essential if a partnership is to be established between the nurse, patient and relatives.

Nursing staff should be given training in interpersonal skills at level one. This training should include the necessary skills to develop a partnership with the patient and the relatives, how to obtain a patient's history in a caring manner and how to prevent violence and deal with aggressive patients. It should also provide the necessary skills to deal appropriately with people who are in need of crisis support or bereavement support.

Wright (1991) identified through a survey of 100 sudden deaths that the time spent by the nurse with relatives of patients who subsequently die ranges from nought to 1 hour (27%), 1–2 hours (46%), and over 2 hours (27%). Wright goes on to say that it would appear that during the period of threat and distress relatives have a heightened or more acute perception of events. Clearly from this work it is essential that A & E nurses receive adequate teaching and training in this area of care. At level three, the nurse should acquire specific counselling skills. Many courses exist and these should be made available so that these nurses become the educators for more junior staff.

Wright suggests that there is a need for specialist helpers to deal with the numerous complexities of human problems and for nurses these problems are part of the whole patient: for some the problems will be minor whereas for others they will be a major part of the patient's focus. Wright adds that nurses cannot be part of the healing process and ignore the psychological problems; their need to respond to these problems is as great as the patient's need for them to be met.

The development of the nurse's role in the care of patients goes beyond just developing their interpersonal skills: it also involves the nurse being the key person in developing the environment that patients and relatives are placed in. The introduction of relatives' sitting rooms, and the use of quiet rooms or chapels within the A & E department are just a few examples of nurses identifying the needs of the client.

Triage

This activity is probably the most important nursing development that has occurred in the UK's A & E departments over the last 10 years. Triage means to sort, pick, select. It originates from the French word 'trier' and has been used not only in the English wool industry but in military medicine for many years. The first major use of triage in military history was in the First World War. It was used to sort the casualties into priority groups for medical aid. The first reference to the use of triage in an A & E department comes from Yale, Newhaven Hospital, USA.

In 1963 triage was used in a non-disaster situation. All patients entering the department were prioritised into one of several categories. Formal triage in the UK appeared in the 1980s. Today it is widely accepted that the most appropriate person to carry out triage is a nurse who has a wide experience and knowledge in A & E nursing. The nursing staff in the A & E department must be trained to undertake triage. Triage is a dynamic process and priorities will alter if the patient's condition changes or other emergencies occur. The nursing staff making these decisions need to have completed an in-house training programme.

This training programme should commence as part of the level one programme. The nurse should be encouraged to observe triage in operation and begin to understand how nursing staff decide on the priority category. Formal in-house training should be included as part of the level two programme. The in-house training package should include an introduction to triage, setting the priority categories and allowing the nurses to discuss the allocation of patients to these categories. The training should also include in-depth patient assessment and lectures. The use of skill stations can be very beneficial.

Triage should be carried out in any clinical area. It comprises a first stage nursing assessment (non-written) which should be conducted immediately the patient arrives in the department. This immediate assessment provides the nurse with the information necessary to decide on an initial priority category, for example, immediate medical intervention or can wait to receive a second stage nursing assessment. The patients' charter standard five supports this system and states clearly, 'The charter standard is that you will be seen immediately and your need for treatment assessed'. The second stage (written nursing assessment) provides a more in-depth understanding of the patient's presenting problem. From this second stage assessment a more accurate priority category can be allocated.

The amount of priority categories used in the A & E department is in the hands of the staff. Most departments use either three or four categories. These can be linked with waiting times and provide an excellent source of information when records are audited. The North East Thames Regional Health Authority in their publication *Accident and Emergency Services: a Guide to Good Practice* (NETRHA 1992) have agreed a priority system which will be used throughout the region to facilitate comparison between departments. The following four priority groups are recommended.

- Priority 1: patients who require immediate attention. This priority is sub-divided into:
- Priority 1a: standby, immediate medical intervention on arrival.
- Priority 1b: must be seen by the medical staff within 15 minutes from arrival.
- Priority 2: must be seen by the medical staff within 1 hour from arrival. Again this group is sub-divided into:
- Priority 2a: need on medical grounds.
- Priority 2b: need on social grounds.
- Priority 3: can safely wait up to 3 hours for medical attention.
- Priority 4: while these can wait indefinitely for treatment, a ceiling of 4 hours has been established.

The allocation of a patient to a priority category must not be based solely on diagnostic coding, such as all fractured toes in one category, but must be based on the assessment of the individual. Children and other vulnerable patients may well be allocated a higher priority. The nurse performing triage is accountable for the decisions made regarding the priority category allocated. It is essential therefore that only a nurse who has completed the local training and has been found competent to assess, identify problems and prioritise patients should be working at the triage desk or performing triage in the clinical area.

The problem-oriented approach

The majority of patients present to the A & E department complaining of a particular problem, for example a wound, an injured arm, or a head injury. Following a nursing assessment other actual or potential problems can be identified. By using the model of nursing the nurse can assess, identify actual and potential problems, set realistic goals, carry out interventions and evaluate the care given. The degree of patient assessment and intervention will be based on the knowledge and skills acquired by the nurse and the local policy. Under the 'extended role' approach this would have comprised a number of listed tasks, for example the nurse may or may not record an ECG, perform a blood test to determine the patient's blood sugar, give oxygen or Entonex without medical approval, or perform wound suturing.

With the publication of *The Scope of Professional Practice* the nursing activities during the assessment and intervention stages of care should be based on the patient's needs and the development programme should reflect this. During the first level programme the nurse will be trained in the correct assessment and intervention of patients presenting with all manner of conditions. Some of these patients will need very little in the way of active procedures during the assessment or intervention stage. Much of the assessment will be based on the nursing history, signs and symptoms and the nurse's interpretation of this information. Other patients will require further procedures such as an assessment of the pulse, blood pressure, ECG, blood sugar, peak flow, neurological status, etc.

The training should allow the nurse to perform an assessment based on the need of the patient, not a list of do's and don'ts. The same applies to intervention: the nurse must acquire the knowledge and skills necessary to intervene based on the patient's needs. This may include the need to support a patient or relative in crisis. It may also include the performance of advanced life-saving skills such as defibrillation, intubation and intravenous cannulation. If appropriate these procedures must be taught as part of the overall training in the care of the patient suffering from chest pain or the overall care of the patient with major injuries. These procedures taught in isolation simply return nursing to the extended task days.

Although throughout the level one training the nurse will be exposed to all types of patients with all manner of human needs, some specific patients need to be highlighted within the programme.

Human behaviour

An understanding of the care of the patient with human behavioural problems is essential. These problems may be of a psychiatric nature or may be the result of an over-consumption of alcohol or drugs. Because of the different types of human behavioural problems which present in the A & E department, and because many of these can be of a psychiatric nature, it is advisable for all departments to have at least one registered mental nurse on the staff. This person should act as a resource and should provide teaching to other staff.

The elderly

The elderly person has very specific needs. These needs will vary between each individual but will normally include the need for the nurse to perform a very detailed social assessment and if the patient is to be discharged there will possibly be a need for the nurse to organise social and nursing support in the community. Walsh (1985a) claims that it is wrong to think of the elderly as the same as everyone else only older. The profound physiological, psychological and sociological changes associated with ageing mean that nurses must consider the elderly as having a unique field of problems that is deserving of special consideration.

Children

Children have needs which include the need for separate waiting and treatment facilities. The nurse must appreciate the special skills required in the nursing of children and must develop the ability to identify non-accidental injury. The nurse must learn how to identify the child that is not deliberately injured but due to inexperienced parents will be at risk if further support from the health visitor is not arranged.

The North East Thames Regional Health Authority (NETRHA) guide recommends that every department should have education programmes for all staff on the needs and care of children. Local policies and procedures should be based on national reports and guidelines. The employment of a registered sick children's nurse (or in future one who has qualified through the child branch of the RN qualification) in the department will provide the staff with a resource and this nurse should provide the teaching and training in the care of the paediatric patient.

The management of patients with major injuries

The Royal College of Surgeons (RCS) has urged action to improve the care of patients with severe injuries (RCS 1988). The National Audit Office has recommended early and continuing improvements to ensure uniformly good provision for care of all severely injured patients and consideration is to be given by the Department of Health and the NHS as to how trauma audit should be carried forward (National Audit Office 1992a, 1992b). A guide to good practice for A & E services (NETRHA 1992) recommends that a minimum of one nurse and one doctor trained to advanced trauma life support level (or the equivalent) should be available 24 hours per day. It also recommends the availability of a trauma team and this team should include trained nurses.

This emphasis on the improvement in trauma management has major implications for nurses working in A & E. Not only must care of the patient with severe injuries be introduced as part of the level one training but this care must be developed through level two and even into level four. The nurse at level one must be taught how to correctly assess the trauma patient. This assessment should be based on the recognised trauma care protocols taught in the advanced trauma care courses.

The assessment must start with the care of the airway and the provision of cervical spine precautions. Once this has been managed, the assessment of the patient's breathing, circulation and neurological status is performed. At any stage, interventions to reduce life threatening conditions are carried out. The nursing assessment continues with an in-depth inspection from head to toe, the nurse identifying injuries and potential injuries. Intervention is based on providing life-support measures, many of which will be taught on the recognised courses.

It is essential at level one that the nurse becomes familiar with all the equipment in the resuscitation room. The nurse should be able not only to operate the equipment safely but also be aware of how to maintain the equipment and how to deal with common problems which can occur. Oxygen administration is an area of concern in many departments. Often the trauma patient is given inadequate oxygen in the belief it may do some harm. Trauma patients need high percentage oxygen and this must be given immediately on arrival by the nurse. At level two nurses should be encouraged to attend one of the national trauma nursing courses. It is also appropriate at level two for nurses to be taught specific life-support techniques through in-house courses. These should include venepuncture and IV cannulation, advanced airway care including intubation, and defibrillation.

Law and ethics

The A & E department is a minefield for legal and ethical issues. The nurse must be taught how to deal with problems that occur on a regular basis. Policies and procedures must be followed when dealing with sudden death, firearms, drugs, violence, etc. The nurse should attend as part of level one training a study day on Law and the Nurse. This study day should address such issues as negligence, accountability, confidentiality and should include legal issues pertaining to the patient in A & E; issues such as the nurse's role in road traffic accident cases, and how and when to summon police help. There should be in-house training to help the nurse deal with the ethical issues which will be encountered. This is especially pertinent in respect of resuscitation, finding illegal substances on patients and dealing with injured patients when a crime may or may not have been committed.

The nurse should be aware of *The Code of Professional Conduct* (UKCC 1992a) and the support leaflet which deals with the subject of confidentiality (UKCC 1987).

Forensic evidence is essential in certain cases and the nurse must be taught how to handle such evidence. Records are often requested by the police. The nurse must know what can and cannot be released and under what circumstances. Because of the nature of the work, the press often make enquiries. The nurse must know how to handle this situation.

Management development

Although the majority of management training is included at levels three and four, it is important that an understanding and appreciation of management issues is introduced from day one. The nurse during the orientation stage must be made aware of the need for a clear management command structure within the department. Most A & E departments are complex and require senior A & E nurses to manage them on a daily basis. The department can be subdivided into identified clinical areas and nurses during level two training should be taught how to manage a clinical area. Irrespective of the process used to deliver care, for example primary or team nursing, the nurse during level two must be taught how to deliver care as the named nurse.

The named nurse, as identified earlier, is one of the patient charter standards. The standard identifies that a named nurse must be responsible for each patient and that nurse will be responsible for the patient's nursing care. Guidance from the patient charter group suggests that the named nurse should be responsible for the patient during the total period the patient requires care. In A & E the nurse responsible for the patient in the resuscitation room should become the named nurse. In the cubicles it should be the team leader, plus or minus other nurses in the area. The triage nurse should be the named nurse for the patients in the waiting room.

Level three should prepare the nurse to start co-ordinating the department on a shift basis. The nurse should be sent on the various management modules, either within the hospital's own staff development structure, or to recognised courses in the local college or university. The nurse should also be taught how to respond and co-ordinate the department during a major incident.

Audit is the systematic critical analysis of the quality of patient care against previously agreed standards. Setting of standards and the nurse's role in audit should be introduced at level one, developed at level two and used as part of the level four programme. The nurse at level four should be taught how to audit the performance of other nurses both concurrent and retrospective. In the A & E department no attempt should be made to separate nursing audit from medical audit; it should be conducted as clinical audit.

The emergency nurse practitioner

Much controversy has surrounded the development of the emergency nurse practitioner in major A & E departments. The first A & E nurse practitioner was established in Oldchurch Hospital, Romford in 1986. This development was as a direct result of a major survey undertaken by the hospital and local Community Health Council. The scheme was introduced to try and reduce the long waiting time experienced by many patients. Two of the key factors in the Oldchurch system were the ability for the emergency nurse practitioner to assess, diagnose, treat and discharge certain patients who were suffering from what were described as minor injuries and to refer patients with potential fractures to the X-ray department before the patient was seen by the doctor.

The activity of a nurse seeing patients, treating and discharging them without reference to a doctor was not new. Many minor casualties, usually in rural areas, have provided this type of service for many years. These departments are normally serviced by local GPs who will attend the patient only if the nursing staff in the department require a medical input to the patient's care.

Following the Oldchurch experience, which showed a reduction in patient waiting time, other departments started to develop this concept. Some departments decided to develop the role by employing A & E nurses specifically to perform this duty at certain times of the day, usually at peak patient attendance times. These nurses have been given job descriptions that identify their role in the department as an emergency nurse practitioner and they are not expected to work in other areas of the department, for example major trolley area or the resuscitation room.

Other departments chose to develop this role in a given number of staff so that the service could be provided on a 24 hour basis. This approach also retained the nurse as a practitioner who would work in any area of the department. The nurse would be allocated the emergency nurse practitioner role for a shift in the same way as other nurses are allocated to areas such as major trolleys or resuscitation. This difference in approach, while not in itself being unacceptable, has caused confusion and to some extent still does. The nurse who is employed as an emergency nurse practitioner and wears a name badge with this title, is in many eyes seen to be different to the nurse who is practising this expanded role but remains in the department as a staff nurse or sister.

Another major problem surrounds the educational requirement for such an expanded role. Should there be a nationally recognised course or should it be based on local needs? Some nurses in the early days of this initiative suggested that simple experience was sufficient; this just added to the confusion and concern that many nurses and doctors were now exhibiting. It also had historical links to the pre-1977 situation and was in most A & E circles totally unacceptable.

Because this new role was first developed during the extended skills era, practitioners had to develop a list of conditions they were permitted to treat without reference to a doctor. Some of these lists reflected the absurdity of the extended role and included many activities that A & E nurses practise as a normal part of their duties. Lists between hospitals varied and often one of the key areas of controversy was the requests by nurses for X-ray examination. The Royal College of Radiologists and Radiographers were opposed to this activity and it was left to local agreement. This situation remains today, although recent research, as yet unpublished, will hopefully change this situation. A study undertaken by the Royal Colleges of Radiologists, Radiographers, and Nursing, and the British Association of A & E Medicine has shown that it is safe for nurses to request X-ray examinations prior to the patient seeing the doctor and it reduces the overall time the patient spends in the department.

The Royal College of Nursing's A & E Association defines the emergency nurse practitioner as,

> 'an A & E nurse who has a sound nursing practice base in all aspects of A & E nursing, with formal post-basic education in holistic assessment, physical diagnosis, prescription of treatment and promotion of health. The emergency nurse practitioner must be a key member of the health care team and directly available to members of the public. He/she must be an autonomous practitioner, able to assess, diagnose, treat and discharge patients without reference to a doctor, but within prearranged guidelines. He/she must be able to make independent referral to other health care professionals.'

NETRHA define an emergency nurse practitioner as an experienced nurse who is allowed, without reference to a doctor, to assess, diagnose, prescribe treatment and discharge patients, whose conditions fall within guidelines set up by the hospital.

These two definitions clearly identify the role of the emergency nurse practitioner. It is clear by these definitions that the role should only be carried out by an A & E nurse who not only has a sound nursing practice base in A & E but also has undertaken some formal post-basic education to equip her with the appropriate skills to practise. It is irrelevant as to how the nurse is employed, for example as an emergency nurse practitioner or as a staff nurse or sister who practises as an emergency nurse practitioner.

My own view is that the development of this role should be included in the development programme and the nurse should undertake the necessary training as part of the level three development. The training for this role should be nationally recognised and should either become a part of the ENB 'Course 3' or should become a separate ENB course. The training should be based around the current programme offered at Southend Hospital. This 4-day package prepares the nurse to practise as an emergency nurse practitioner. It includes biological sciences, behavioural sciences, developments in care, professional and personal development and ethics and law. Lectures cover head, ENT, eye and facio-maxillary injuries; wound care and burns; history taking; medico-legal implications; and assessment and examination of ankles and feet, wrists and hands. Practical sessions include suturing and plastering, health promotion, observation with the nurse practitioner and A & E senior house officer. The nurse must also practise as a supervised practitioner and this session is audited as part of the course.

Education and research

All nurses have an obligation to support and teach their colleagues. This can only be performed effectively if they themselves are taught how to teach. At level two the nurse should be taught how to act as mentor to student nurses and junior staff in the department. The nurse should complete a recognised course in teaching and assessing. The use of research information in current practice should be encouraged at all development levels.

At level two the nurse should obtain more formal understanding of research and how the use of research can enhance practice in A & E care. Kirby (1990) describes how a much wider use of available nursing research can be readily applied to nursing practice as a means of improving the quality of care to patients and their relatives. As part of level four the nurse should be taught how to undertake research within the department.

Our medical colleagues see A & E as an essential area for medical research; nurses must not be left behind. Level four is aimed at developing the now expert A & E nurse into an A & E clinical specialist. To achieve this requires the nurse to develop expertise in one or more sub-specialities within the A & E nursing field. Examples of such clinical development are care of the child, bereavement care and trauma care. It is also essential at this level for the nurse to be able to conduct nursing research. (For a summary of levels of training see Appendix IV in this volume.)

Nurses should be encouraged to teach medical staff and this should be formally recognised. Teaching in A & E must be team-based and not discipline-based. Annual and ongoing appraisal should be part of the educational system and each nurse should have their individual development programme reviewed and updated.

Conclusion

The expanding role of the nurse in the A & E department must occur in direct response to the needs of the patient and the relatives. No additional task should be undertaken unless it benefits the client. The development programme described in this chapter is based on this belief and links comfortably with *The Scope of Professional Practice*. To quote Moores (1992):

> '*The Code of Professional Conduct* and *The Scope of Professional Practice* begin a process which affords all practitioners the opportunity to develop and use their education, skills and knowledge to maximise their contribution to patient care and at the same time achieve the highest level of personal fulfilment.'

References

Ashcroft J. (1992) Rising to the challenge. *Nursing Times* **88**, 30.
Blythin P. (1988) Triage in the UK. *Nursing*, 3 November, 16.
Cliff K. (1982) Where the nurse fits in. *Nursing Mirror*, 12 May, 22.
Cole A. (1986) Specialist support from above. *Nursing Times*, 14 May, 18.
Department of Health and Social Security (1977) *The extending role of the nurse.* Health Circular HC(77)22. DHSS, London.

Department of Health (1989) *A Strategy for Nursing.* DoH Nursing Division, London.

Department of Health (1992) *The Patients' Charter.* DoH, London.

Eaves D. (1987) Why we should care in A & E. *Nursing Times* **83**, 31.

Jones G. (1984) Code rendered pointless. *Nursing Mirror*, 12 December, **159**, 12.

Jones G. (1986) Behind the times. *Nursing Times*, 15 October, 30.

Jones G. (1988) Top priority. *Nursing Standard*, 12 November, **3**, 28.

Jones G. (1990) *Accident and Emergency Nursing: A Structured Approach.* Faber and Faber, London.

Kirby M. (1990) Research application in A & E departments. *Nursing*, 26 April, **4**, 20.

Moores Y. (1992) Setting new boundaries. *Nursing Times*, 9 September, **88**, 28.

National Audit Office (1992a) *NHS Accident and Emergency Departments in England.* NAO, London.

National Audit Office (1992b) *NHS Accident and Emergency Departments in Scotland.* NAO, London.

North East Thames Regional Health Authority (1992) *Accident and Emergency Services: A Guide to Good Practice for Providers.* NETRHA, London.

NHS Management Executive (1992) *Hours of Work of Doctors in Training. Making the Best Use of the Skills of Nurses and Midwives.* DoH, London.

Royal College of Surgeons (1988) *The Management of Patients with Major Injuries.* RCS, London.

Salvage J. (1986) The frontier spirit. *Senior Nurse*, 27 February, **2**, 1.

United Kingdom Central Council for Nursing, Midwifery and Health Visiting (1987) *Confidentiality.* UKCC, London.

United Kingdom Central Council for Nursing, Midwifery and Health Visiting (1990) *Report of the Post-Registration Education & Practice Project (PREPP).* UKCC, London.

United Kingdom Central Council for Nursing, Midwifery and Health Visiting (1992a) *Code of Professional Conduct.* UKCC, London.

United Kingdom Central Council for Nursing, Midwifery and Health Visiting (1992b) *The Scope of Professional Practice*, UKCC, London.

Walsh M. (1985a) The special branch. *Senior Nurse*, 6 February, **2**, 11.

Walsh M. (1985b) *Accident and Emergency Nursing: A New Approach.* Heinemann, London.

Wright B. (1986) *Caring in crisis.* Churchill Livingstone, London.

Wright B. (1991) *Sudden death.* Churchill Livingstone, London.

Chapter 12
Health Care Assistants and Accountability

Introduction

The expansion of the nursing role will, within the health care hierarchy, have an upward impact – on the medical profession, and a downward impact – on support workers. Indeed, the expanding role of the nurse is just one dimension of radical changes in the delivery of health care, and cannot be fully understood without taking into account changes in the role of the other occupational groups involved. In this chapter we shall look at the 'health care assistant' (HCA) and try to come to grips with this role in the context of the expanding scope of nursing practice.

The development of HCAs is very much tied up with the proliferation of national vocational qualifications (NVQs). The NVQ movement in health care may perhaps be seen as a kind of 'semi-professionalisation' of support staff, following in the wake of the professionalisation of nursing. It is part and parcel of the wider phenomenon of the professionalisation of society and a reflection of the current public policy of subjecting work to analysis, measurable standards and outcomes on the assumption that public welfare delivery is accessible to an industrial model.

Indeed, NVQs were first introduced in the industrial and commercial sectors of the economy, being already established in over 250 areas of work outside health. NVQs have been described as a 'new approach to management' and a 'tool' by which managers can draw up business plans. One manager has emphasised that 'in future purchasers will be asking units to say how much time has been spent training, to what level are people being trained' (National Health Service Training Directorate 1991). There are, of course, dangers in subjecting welfare to a managerial model designed for industry and commerce, although we shall not enter into that debate here (Hunt 1991).

HCAs have to be taken in economic context. It has become apparent that the government policy is to cut down on nursing staff and nurse educators. Intakes of nursing students are decreasing dramatically and will continue to drop, even if we consider only demographic trends. Student nurses pursuing Project 2000 courses are supernumerary in the workplace. Meanwhile, patients and potential patients are ever increasing. The question arises – who will be looking after the patients and clients? There are widespread concerns that qualified nursing staff will become 'resource managers' while HCAs do the basic nursing. Are HCAs merely a cheap alternative to nurses? Does the development of HCAs threaten nursing posts? It is not clear at present how far such concerns are justified.

Who will nurse?

Allman has posed a central question about current changes in the delivery of nursing care.

'So far, however, there has been insufficient attention to a fundamental impact that degrees in nursing and the thinking behind them could have for provision of services and free movement at European Community level. If the entire profession of nursing goes 'up market' in terms of its outlook and function, it will leave a vacuum behind it. In over-simple language, who will do the bedside nursing if today's trained nurse becomes an organiser, coordinator and planner rather than the provider of direct and personal patient care?' (Allman 1993, p. 38)

Nursing auxiliaries and assistants have, of course, worked alongside SENs and RGNs for many years. These were often the people assisting clients with fundamental care and the activities of daily living – helping someone to wash and dress, eat and drink, move around, urinate, etc. They are often on the spot if significant changes occur in the patient's condition and alert the qualified staff or assist the patient until help comes.

HCAs will be undertaking many of the tasks previously undertaken routinely by nursing auxiliaries, and some tasks undertaken from time to time by SENs and RGNs. For example, they will be expected to detect signs of pressure sores and take action to minimise such sores, enable clients to maintain personal hygiene and appearances, help with dressing in a manner relevant to the patient's medical condition, assist clients with eating and drinking in a safe fashion, help control infection, assist clients to use toilets, assist in maintaining a comfortable position for the patient consistent with the plan of care, and assist in taking blood pressures and temperatures and collecting of urine samples.

From a managerial point of view a HCA stands outside the traditional NHS employment structure. From the perspective of professional nursing a HCA is:

'A member of staff in health care who has been appointed to a post after a skill mix review or reprofiling exercise whose post does not match any Whitley Council job description. The pay and conditions of health care assistants will be determined locally.' (RCN 1992)

Although support workers are generally mature individuals with valuable experience and have much to offer they are sometimes treated as if their contribution is of little consequence. They have been and still are a neglected group of workers and unfortunately nurses have not always been helpful in developing their abilities.

There are both potential benefits and some dangers in the training and re-training of support workers under the framework of the National Council for Vocational Qualifications (NCVQ) and the Scottish Vocational Educational Council (SCOTVEC.) A lot depends on what *nurses* make of the new opportunities. The expansion of the role of the nurse should mean a new and positive attitude and working relationship with support workers.

For the better?

Nurses are now involved directly in the training of HCAs (some of them already nursing auxiliaries). Since the HCA obtains their NVQ in the workplace principally on the basis of being able to *perform* according to standards set within the workplace itself, the qualified nursing staff now have the opportunity to define what is essentially 'nursing' and what is 'health care assistance'. We shall consider this in greater detail in what follows.

This is an excellent opportunity for nurses to act as advocates of patients, ensuring that they receive the kind of nursing care that they themselves would like to receive. It is an opportunity for nurses to expand their role and enhance their skills in *nursing care,* by taking full advantage of the more skilful and committed assistance they can expect from NVQ-qualified HCAs.

In the Project 2000 Report HCAs (referred to as 'aides') are conceived as workers who will free up more time for nursing judgement and action by executing the more simple and routine tasks (UKCC 1986). Thus the HCA is not a type of nurse at all.

There is already evidence that NVQ training is good for the status and self-esteem of support workers, and by the same token good for patient care:

'Those who have undergone training and assessment have responded with considerable enthusiasm and motivation. Managers have noted a positive change of attitude in a number of staff. The opportunity to obtain a qualification recognising their skills and ability has given HCAs increased job satisfaction. They seem to feel more valued as part of the team. The training has also highlighted the considerable wealth of experience and ability which HCAs possess. The measurement of HCAs' competence and skills against national performance standards is seen by many managers as providing an assurance of improved quality of care to patients and clients.' (Evans & Young 1993)

For the worse?

A concern with cost, professional status and staff recruitment under present demographic and economic conditions must have been taken into account by the Project 2000 Report authors in their deliberations on the role of HCAs. They were trying to make the best of a difficult economic and labour situation while seeking ways of improving nursing care. This is perfectly in accord with the emphasis the Report puts on patients' rights and nursing autonomy.

However, there may be a disparity between the hopeful vision of Project 2000 and the market ideology and objectives of the 1980s and 1990s (Hunt 1992a).

The Project 2000 Report denies that nurses will be taken further away from patients, casting them in a merely supervisory role while the new non-nursing cadre of HCAs do the nursing (UKCC 1986, pp. 39–40, 43). It would be very wrong to suggest that the creation of an 'army of the unqualified' supervised by hands-off nurses is the intention of the Report. Nevertheless one has to ask what the consequences will be of implementing the plan in the actual circumstances of a Government policy preoccupied above all else with the reduction of public expenditure by freeing up market forces.

In the ideology of the New Right nursing itself is suspect, for it is viewed perhaps as a somewhat patronising and nannying activity which subverts the initiative of people who should really be supported by family and community (David 1986). In these terms a reduced health care system in which basic care is delivered by a large number of low-cost non-professionals would be seen as a 'cost-effective' alternative.

In other words, whatever the intentions of the Project 2000 plan for

HCAs, it may be appropriated by the new commercial management and distorted to meet its own ends.

The Report suggests that such a distortion would have implications for practice which would stand 'in contravention of the UKCC Code of Professional Conduct' (UKCC 1986, p. 43). However, it would appear that at present Government, health authorities or hospital trust management are not very inclined to change administrative structures and the law so as to enable nurses to put the Code into effect. Indeed, it would not be surprising if the statutory bodies and the Government end up on a collision course. Certainly some health carers who have dared to live by their professional ethics and have voiced concerns about standards have found themselves victimised.

Who will be accountable and how?

The UKCC has made quite clear in section 23 of *The Scope of Professional Practice* document how nurses and HCAs relate to one another (see Appendix I in this volume). HCAs must 'work under the direction and supervision' of the registered nurses, midwives and health visitors whom they are assisting; must 'not be allowed to work beyond their level of competence'; and the registered practitioner remains accountable for 'assessment, planning and standards of care and for determining the activity of their support staff' (UKCC 1992).

While nurses and doctors are subject to statutory regulation, support workers are not. HCAs are not registered by the UKCC or any similar body and are not currently eligible for membership of the Royal College of Nursing. The NVQ movement may be seen as a back-up system in the absence of such regulation, developing occupational standards and qualifications as a recognition of competence to practise.

The question of the accountability of HCAs may be viewed from the point of view of their competence, their responsibility and the authority which they have or do not have.

Who is responsible for the mistakes, lapses in duty of care, and negligence of the HCA? Is the HCA personally responsible? Is the nurse? Is the employer or the health authority? The HCA is subject to many of the same legal sanctions as any health care worker – the civil and criminal law, and contractual obligations to the employer. However, in the absence of a statutory regulatory body the HCA is not accountable in the way a nurse is accountable under the provisions of the 1979 and 1992 Acts (HMSO 1979, 1992). It is perhaps partly due to this fact that many nurses worry that they will have to carry the can for any shortcomings of the HCA working under their direction.

Acting outside competence

What if a HCA goes beyond their competence, carrying out something which a nurse ordered them to do? This situation is in many ways similar to that in which a nurse does what a doctor tells them even though it is outside their competence. Both the doctor and the nurse are wrong. (Dimond has discussed related issues in Chapter 4.) In the present case both the nurse and the HCA would be wrong, and the nurse could among other things face a UKCC disciplinary hearing while the HCA would face a hearing internal to the place of employment.

Admittedly, the danger is that under pressure HCAs will feel they have no alternative but to do what they are told, just as nurses often feel this in relation to doctors' instructions. While nurses have blown the whistle on intolerable situations such as these, it would not be surprising if in the future HCAs do so.

The new HCA role is actually meant to *enhance* the accountability of the nurse. That is, the Project 2000 Report envisages a situation in which the assistance of competent HCAs will enable nurses to practise more autonomously and responsibly. As we have seen, the Report states that a merely supervisory nursing role would contravene the accountability which nurses have imposed on them by statute.

Nurses can be held responsible for some blunders of HCAs, but not for every blunder as a matter of principle. In theory at least, the nurses cannot be held blameworthy for some lapse in an HCA's duty of care – say incorrectly lifting a patient – if it can be shown that the HCA had been adequately trained and assessed and properly directed and monitored by the delegating nurse.

It is useful perhaps to keep in mind a distinction between *system-responsibility* and *action-responsibility*. Thus the nurse in charge (the ward sister, for example) could only be held directly and wholly responsible for a wrongful action on the part of the HCA where that action was the outcome of a wrongly designed, implemented, monitored or directed system of work. At a lower level, the delegating nurse could only be wholly responsible where that action was the outcome of deficient supervision, monitoring or direction – and even here the delegating nurse cannot be expected to supervise every single action for that would defeat the point of employing HCAs. The nurse is expected to monitor in general, and to assure that the HCA has shown a general competence to carry out the task in question.

It would clearly be against natural justice to lay down as a general principle that the ward manager or delegating nurse has to be held responsible for everything the HCA could possibly do wrong. There are many possible scenarios in which the HCA would be held solely responsible and the nurse exonerated. In practice, admittedly, the relevant nurses would always come under scrutiny where there were lapses and there might be a burden on them to show that there had been proper monitoring and direction. This is a burden which goes with the authority that the delegating nurse has, a burden which all nurses will have to accept if they wish to expand their role.

Analogously, the health authority for example carries an even heavier burden in cases of litigation and might have to accept vicarious liability.

HCA role extension?

The question also arises of whether the role of the HCA will be susceptible to extension or even expansion. Which competencies would be considered as 'extended' in the case of HCAs – blood sugar or blood pressure monitoring? At the moment it would appear that the HCA role is quite clearly delimited in terms of tasks but it remains true that there will almost certainly be pressure under existing conditions to extend the HCA role and that it will be necessary for hospital policies in this regard to be explicit (written down) and sufficiently detailed (Hunt 1992b).

Many difficulties concerning the accountability of HCAs can be circumvented by greater attention to job descriptions and contracts, with greater detail about competencies, duties and rights, and mechanisms of accountability (Hunt 1992b).

Resources

This question is tied up with that of the availability of resources. Are there sufficient nurses, and the right kind, on duty? Are there sufficient numbers and the right kind of HCA on duty? The RCN has noted the resource problem:

'The nurse must be satisfied that the available support workers are competent to give the nursing care required and must be able to give adequate supervision. If not, the nurse must take action to safeguard patients by informing those who control the supply of staff to the team.' (RCN 1992)

Arbitration

The ward manager will generally be the person that the HCA is primarily accountable to. The ward manager is responsible for setting competencies, ensuring that HCAs were adequately trained, assessing, monitoring and general guidance. In cases of misunderstanding and dispute it would be fair for the HCA to have a relatively independent party to appeal to. If HCAs are not to lose the goodwill and enthusiasm that many currently have for their work this is absolutely essential. In a hospital setting the site coordinator for HCAs might be the appropriate person for such an arbitrating role (Hunt 1992b).

Given the hierarchical structure of the health service however, it would currently be very difficult in practice for a dissatisfied HCA to take matters to a doctor or manager, although it is our view that this should be regarded as perfectly acceptable in some circumstances. Certainly, established grievance procedures should be as accessible to HCAs as to any other member of staff.

Advocacy

While it is well established, if still somewhat controversial, that nurses are advocates for their patients, not much thought has been given to HCAs as advocates. But given their hands-on and intimate relationship with patients and clients it is obvious that the HCA has a duty to listen to patients, understand their wishes and difficulties and take appropriate action within their competence, and where matters fall outside their competence to report matters to the nurses. Indeed, core NVQ units already stress the attainment of dispositions such as being ready to, 'Contribute to the protection of individuals from abuse', 'Contribute to the ongoing support of clients and others significant to them', 'Contribute to the health, safety and security of individuals and their environment'.

Communication

Effective health care requires team-work and a 'partnership' approach. The Government has insisted that patients have a 'named nurse'. This provides another opportunity for nurses to use their unique skills, because they are the carers who will be coordinating and developing a key relationship with the client. It is the qualified nurse with their awareness of clients' needs and their in-depth knowledge and communication skills who will have to use this to talk to the multidisciplinary team, clients' relatives, other colleagues and agencies who they come into contact with.

The nurse needs to understand and speak to other professionals, the HCAs and the patients/clients in different language frames, sometimes acting as a kind of interpreter. The nurse is at the forefront, so needs to be flexible, versatile, creative and accountable as a practitioner.

The training of health care assistants

We think it is important that nursing staff and nurse educators whole-heartedly take on the role of training HCAs and fully understand what is required. If they do not then they might find that others take over this training role, putting the profession in further jeopardy.

While HCAs are not now strictly required to have any formal training or to hold any recognised qualification, a wide range of NVQs at different levels has been introduced for them.

It is interesting that while the UKCC's 'Scope' document attempts to liberate nurses from certification of tasks and allow them freedom of development in skills without a preoccupation for national consistency in competencies (see Chapter 8), the NVQ movement is doing the direct opposite for support workers.

National vocational qualifications

In September 1992, Tim Yeo MP, Health Minister responsible for Community Care, inaugurated 20 new NVQs for health and social care support staff. The NVQ titles are:

- Developmental Care
- Direct Care
- Domiciliary Support
- Residential/Hospital Support
- Post-Natal Care
- Special Care Needs
- Promoting Independence
- Supported Living
- Rehabilitative Care
- Continuing Care
- Supportive Long Term Care
- Terminal Care
- Acute Care
- Acute Care (Children)
- Clinic and Outpatient Care
- Substance Use
- Support and Protection
- Self and Environmental Management Skills
- Mental Health Care
- Mobility and Movement

This initiative opens the door to formal qualifications, tested in the work environment, for about 250 000 staff.

'The twenty qualifications offer a far greater choice than the original three health care support worker and two residential, domiciliary and day care (RPDC) qualifications (on which they are based). The range of wards now available reflect varying care settings from hospitals and outpatient clinics to residential homes, community settings and clients' own homes. They also cover staff working in support of different professional groups (nurses, midwives, physiotherapists, occupational therapists, social workers, care home owners) and working with differing levels of supervision' (National Health Service Training Directorate 1993).

The NCVQ is responsible for the establishment of the NVQ framework and for ensuring quality in the qualifications accredited within it. This body has overall responsibility for quality assurance, while the awarding bodies have to ensure quality and must approve centres to carry out assessment. Approval is not to be given unless a potential centre can show that it can provide adequately for training and appointing both assessors and internal verifiers. At the same time awarding bodies must recruit external verifiers who will check on the quality assurance systems and provide reports by which national consistency in standards can be achieved.

The general idea of the NVQ is to formalise the skills and experience that thousands of workers obtain working in the interstices of the recognised professions. Support workers obtain NVQs by demonstrating their competence as measured against a set of nationally agreed performance standards. These standards are not drawn up by the NCVQ, although it provides a guiding framework, but by the professionals working in the various areas of care – staff working in the NHS, local government and the voluntary and private sectors. Draft standards are tested within the working environment and are endorsed by managers, trade unions, professional bodies and staff representatives.

NVQs incorporate the assessment of *performance* as well as an evaluation of knowledge and understanding, and the award of such a qualification is independent of the mode of learning, 'That is to say it should not specify a particular programme of learning or period of time as prerequisites to attainment' (NCVQ 1988).

Training in the nursing environment

To understand the concerns of qualified staff in relation to HCAs one has to look at the historical background of support work. These workers were never required to have formal training or recognised qualifications. There was no comprehensive, organised training for them. As a result training was fragmented. In some areas they received some form of training and in others they did not. The same applied to the level of supervision. At times support workers took on tasks beyond their job descriptions. At other times they were told they could not perform those tasks because only student nurses and qualified staff could do so. It often depended on who was in charge. Overstretching and deskilling often took place.

While many support workers were valued within the context of the multi-disciplinary team others felt and still feel undervalued. In the hierarchical structure that exists in health care this gives some qualified staff a sense of power and also secures their position because they have this barrier which protects them from exposing their own inadequacies and insecurities.

However, in order to fully integrate nursing support workers the qualified nurse must be satisfied that the HCA within the team is competent for the work required. It is no longer good enough to say 'I know they can do the work alright'. The NCVQ requires proof of competency and evidence to support this. This is something entirely new for qualified staff.

To repeat, the NCVQ approach to training means that nurses have the opportunity to give shape to the role of HCAs, to set the standards they expect of them, and thereby define their accountability.

What better way to manage support staff than by clearly indicating what is expected of them and precisely defining their role? NVQ training goes hand in hand with a certain managerial context. Managers will be expected to undertake functional mapping, establish the required skill mix for each nursing situation, promoting high standards of patient care to be maintained and monitored through an effective quality assurance system.

Preparation of qualified staff

The emphasis is on workplace training which requires a comprehensive understanding by trained staff of what is involved in the training of HCAs and what is required of other members of staff in clinical settings. In some hospitals, for example, wards and departments have on their staff a significant number of people who have undertaken the course in 'Training and Assessing in Clinical Practice' (ENB998). Two-day workshops have proved useful and convenient in informing staff who will be assessing HCAs in training, ensuring that in each area where a trainee is present there is a suitable supervisor/assessor who is knowledgeable about the NVQ System and Assessment Process and experienced in their occupational area (Hunt 1992b).

Assessment of competence

The question about accountability usually turns out to be one about ensuring the *competence* of HCAs. It is also about the added responsibilities that qualified staff have to adopt in order to offer support workers in their area a NVQ training.

The training of HCAs involves continuous assessment in the workplace until the trainee is competent. It requires qualified staff to ensure that standards are maintained and that performance is measured against set criteria. When competence has been achieved the assessor signs off the necessary standard stating that they have assessed the HCAs and found them to be competent in a particular unit of care, e.g. personal hygiene and grooming.

NVQs require qualified staff to sign a statement of competence for health care assistants. The job descriptions of HCAs are important. Functional mapping is being undertaken in health authorities; skill mix review and job re-profiling allow the employers to move towards roles which allow better use of staff resources and ensure that professional competencies and specialities are used to the best effect.

Nurses have always supervised student nurses and other co-workers depending on their status in the nursing hierarchy. They might have written reports on their colleagues or given verbal reports. Qualified staff assessed nurses in the clinical area and recorded performance. Qualified staff were engaged with learner nurses and reported on their progress after the allocated time to the clinical area ended. So what is required in NVQ assessment is not completely alien to registered nurses. Responsibilities include the following assessment tasks:

(1) Conduct an initial assessment to determine the competencies which an individual may already possess.
(2) Agree an individual plan of action with staff.
(3) Ensure provision is made available for candidates to acquire competencies.
(4) Give feedback to the HCA and review progress.
(5) See that sufficient evidence is collected.
(6) Ensure that evidence is judged against the performance criteria and range statements for each of the elements of competence.
(7) Ensure that the candidates' achievements are agreed and recorded in the assessment books.

HCAs usually work in a multidisciplinary setting, so that a number of staff will have supervised them and given evidence about their performance.

If the performance criteria are not met then this is discussed with the candidates concerned and a new plan of action devised. If for any reason the candidate does not subsequently perform their job to the required standard then, provided all the rules have been observed, this does not challenge their role as an assessor but rather highlights a problem with the employee which management has to deal with.

If after this action has been taken the candidate does not work to the required standard, and has been directed and supervised adequately, then the candidate has failed to fulfil the role as agreed in the job description and the disciplinary procedure may be invoked.

If, however, the registered staff failed to use the standards and measure performance against the performance criteria, and did not notice (or noticed but did not act on the fact) that the HCA was not maintaining standards, then they could be held liable, or this could be construed as neglect of duty since this may put the client in jeopardy. For example, an assessing nurse may culpably fail to observe, through not taking the trouble to check, that an HCA fails to follow the principles of cross-infection by omitting to wash hands after attending to a client or by not disposing of contaminated material in a safe and proper manner.

Evidence

Evidence is produced during the normal working day. HCAs are measured against the performance criteria as stated in the NVQ Standards. As most HCAs work in teams or have a supervisor or named nurse in charge of each shift, evidence is also collected from mentors and other members of the team who work alongside the HCA and others observing them at work.

A majority of HCAs are mature candidates with a varied experience of life. The testimony of those who have witnessed this experience in action is also of great value.

HCAs are also asked to keep a diary of the work they perform and relate it to the endorsements in the NVQ level being undertaken. This demonstrates their understanding of what they are doing and how to apply a range of standards to the work. Underpinning knowledge is continually being assessed in the workplace. HCAs need to demonstrate their competence in communicating with clients and staff, their interpersonal relationships, and the manner in which they record and report back to staff. Evidence of competence is also obtained by direct oral questioning and by completion of assignments.

Conclusion

The development of a large body of HCAs, with vocational qualifications, is both an opportunity for the advancement of nursing care and a potential danger to the future of nursing. It can either enhance nursing autonomy and freedom of judgement for the benefit of patients and clients, or it can put nursing at a greater distance from patients and clients while a large underpaid non-professional workforce struggles with a new regime of tasks and procedures.

Which of these potentials is realised depends to a very great extent on what the nursing profession itself makes of the situation as it expands its scope of practice. Expanding the scope of practice is not about creating more of the same, but about deepening what is best in nursing.

References

Allman S. (1993) 1993 and beyond. In *Nursing: The European Dimension* (eds S. Quinn & S. Russell). Scutari, London.

David M. (1986) Moral and maternal: the family in the right. In *The Ideology of the New Right* (ed. R. Levitas). Polity Press, Cambridge.

Evans W. & Young G. (1993) *Queen Charlotte's College's approach to measuring competence*. Internal Paper, Queen Charlotte's College of Health Care, London.

HMSO (1979, 1992) *Nurses, Midwives and Health Visitors Act*. HMSO, London.

Hunt G. (1991) *Nursing, patient choice and the NHS reforms*. Occasional Paper: Fourth Annual Celebrity Lecture. The National Board for Nursing, Midwifery and Health Visiting for Northern Ireland, Belfast.

Hunt G. (1992a) Project 2000 – ethics, ambivalence and ideology. In *Project 2000 – The Teachers Speak* (eds O. Slevin & M. Buckenham). Campion Press, Edinburgh.

Hunt G. (1992b) Report on a workshop on accountability and the HCA. Internal Paper. Queen Charlotte's College of Health Care, London. Contributors to the workshop convened by the National Centre for Nursing & Midwifery Ethics were Denise Bristow, Winnie Evans, Maggie Hall, Geoff Hunt, Ruth Lallmohamed, Lyn Paton, and Heather Thomas.

National Council for Vocational Qualifications (1988) *Introducing NVQs, implications for education and training. NCVQ Information Leaflet No. 2*. NCVQ, London.

National Health Service Training Directorate (1991) NVQs in the Health Service (Video). NHSTD, Bristol.

National Health Service Training Directorate (1993) *Update No. 5*. NHSTD, Bristol.

Royal College of Nursing (1992) The role of the support worker within the professional nursing team. *Issues in Nursing and Health* **15**. RCN, London.

United Kingdom Council for Nursing, Midwifery and Health Visiting (1986) *Project 2000: A New Preparation for Practice*. UKCC, London.

United Kingdom Council for Nursing, Midwifery and Health Visiting (1992) *The Scope of Professional Practice*. UKCC, London.

Appendices

Appendix I
The Scope of Professional Practice
A UKCC Position Statement

Introduction

(1) The practice of nursing, midwifery and health visiting requires the application of knowledge and the simultaneous exercise of judgement and skill. Practice takes place in a context of continuing change and development. Such change and development may result from advances in research leading to improvements in treatment and care, from alterations to the provision of health and social care services, as a result of changes in local policies and as a result of new approaches to professional practice. Practice must, therefore, be sensitive, relevant and responsive to the needs of individual patients and clients and have the capacity to adjust, where and when appropriate, to changing circumstances.

(2) Education and experience form the foundation on which nurses, midwives and health visitors exercise judgement and skill, these, naturally, being developed and refined over time. The range of responsibilities which fall to individual nurses, midwives and health visitors should be related to their personal experience, education and skill. This range of responsibilities is described here as the 'scope of professional practice' and this paper sets out the Council's principles on which any adjustment to the scope of professional practice should be based. The contents of this paper are as follows:

List of Contents

Education for Professional Practice

(3) Just as practice must remain dynamic, sensitive, relevant and responsive to the changing needs of patients and clients, so too must education for practice. Pre-registration education prepares nurses, midwives and health visitors for safe practice at the point of registration. The pre-registration curriculum will continue to

change over time to absorb relevant changes in care as advances are made. Pre-registration education is, therefore, a foundation for professional practice and a means of equipping nurses, midwives and health visitors with the necessary knowledge and skills to assume responsibility as registered practitioners. This foundation education alone, however, cannot effectively meet the changing and complex demands of the range of modern health care. Post-registration education equips practitioners with additional and more specialist skills necessary to meet the special needs of patients and clients. There is a broad range of post-registration provision and the Council regards adequate and effective provision of quality education as a pre-requisite of quality care.

Registration and the Code of Professional Conduct for the Nurse, Midwife and Health Visitor

(4)   The act of registration by the Council confers on individual nurses, midwives and health visitors the legal right to practise and to use the title 'registered'. From the point of registration, each practitioner is subject to the Council's Code of Professional Conduct and accountable for his or her practice and conduct. The Code provides a statement of the values of the professions and establishes the framework within which practitioners practise and conduct themselves. The act of registration and the expectations stated in the Code are central to the Council's key role in regulating the standards of the professions in the interest of patients and clients and of society as a whole.

(5)   Once registered, each nurse, midwife and health visitor remains subject to the Code and ultimately accountable to the Council for his or her actions and omissions. This position applies regardless of the employment circumstances and regardless of whether or not individuals are actively engaged in practice. This position will only change if the decision is made by the Council (through clearly established legal processes related to professional misconduct or unfitness to practise due to illness) to remove a name from the Council's register. This reflects the key, central role which the registration process plays in maintaining standards in the public interest. On the specific question of employment of nurses in the personal social services in general and the residential care sector in particular, the Council recognises that there are ambiguities. These are addressed in paragraphs 20 and 21 of this paper.

The Code of Professional Conduct and the Scope of Professional Practice

(6)   The Code includes a number of explicit clauses which relate to changes to the scope of practice in nursing, midwifery and health visiting. These clauses are:
   'As a registered nurse, midwife or health visitor you are personally accountable for your practice and, in the exercise of your professional accountability, must:
   (1)   act always in such a manner as to promote and safeguard the interests and well-being of patients and clients;
   (2)   ensure that no action or omission on your part, or within your sphere of responsibility, is detrimental to the interests, condition or safety of patients and clients;
   (3)   maintain and improve your professional knowledge and competence;
   (4)   acknowledge any limitations in your knowledge and competence and decline any duties or responsibilities unless able to perform them in a safe and skilled manner;'

(7)   The Code, therefore, provides a firm bedrock upon which decisions about adjustments to the scope of professional practice can be made. There are, however, important distinctions relating to the scope of practice in nursing, in midwifery and

in health visiting. These are described in the paragraphs that follow the Council's principles for adjusting the scope of practice. These principles apply to the practice of nursing, midwifery and health visiting addressed later in this paper and to any application of complementary or alternative and other therapies by nurses, midwives or health visitors.

Principles for adjusting the Scope of Practice

(8)   Although the practices of nursing, midwifery and health visiting differ widely, the same principles apply to the scope of practice in each of these professions. The following principles are based upon the Council's Code of Professional Conduct and, in particular, on the emphasis which the Code places upon knowledge, skill, responsibility and accountability. The principles which should govern adjustments to the scope of professional practice are those which follow.

(9)   The registered nurse, midwife or health visitor:
  9.1   must be satisfied that each aspect of practice is directed to meeting the needs and serving the interests of the patient or client;
  9.2   must endeavour always to achieve, maintain and develop knowledge, skill and competence to respond to those needs and interests;
  9.3   must honestly acknowledge any limits of personal knowledge and skill and take steps to remedy any relevant deficits in order effectively and appropriately to meet the needs of patients and clients;
  9.4   must ensure that any enlargement or adjustment of the scope of personal professional practice must be achieved without compromising or fragmenting existing aspects of professional practice and care and that the requirements of the Council's Code of Professional Conduct are satisfied throughout the whole area of practice;
  9.5   must recognise and honour the direct or indirect personal accountability borne for all aspects of professional practice and
  9.6   must, in serving the interests of patients and clients and the wider interests of society, avoid any inappropriate delegation to others which compromise those interests.

(10)   These principles for practice should enhance trust and confidence within a health care team and promote further the important collaborative work between medical and nursing, midwifery and health visiting practitioners upon which good practice and care depends.

(11)   The Council recognises that care by registered nurses, midwives and health visitors is provided in health care, social care and domestic settings. Patients and clients require skilled care from registered practitioners and support staff require direction and supervision from these same practitioners. These matters are directly concerned with standards of care. This paper, therefore, also addresses the matter of the 'identified' practitioner, practice in the personal social services and residential care sector and support for professional practice.

The Scope and 'Extended Practice' of Nursing

(12)   The practice of nursing has traditionally been based on the premise that pre-registration education equips the nurse to perform at a certain level and to encompass a particular range of activities. It is also based on the premise that any widening of that range and enhancement of the nurse's practice requires 'official' extension of that role by certification.

(13)   The Council considers that the terms 'extended' or 'extending' roles which have been

associated with this system are no longer suitable since they limit, rather than extend, the parameters of practice. As a result, many practitioners have been prevented from fulfilling their potential for the benefit of patients. The Council also believes that a concentration on 'activities' can detract from the importance of holistic nursing care. The Council has therefore determined the principles set out in paragraphs 8 to 10 inclusive to provide the basis for ensuring that practice remains dynamic and is able readily and appropriately to adjust to meet changing care needs.

(14) The reality is that the practice of nursing, and education for that practice, will continue to be shaped by developments in care and treatment, and by other events which influence it. This equally applies to midwifery and health visiting. **In order to bring into proper focus the professional responsibility and consequent accountability of individual practitioners, it is the Council's principles for practice rather than certificates for tasks which should form the basis for adjustments to the scope of practice.**

The Scope of Midwifery Practice

(15) The position in relation to midwifery practice is set out in the Council's Midwife's Code of Practice. This indicates that it is the individual midwife's responsibility to maintain and develop the competence which she has acquired during her training, recognising the sphere of practice in which she is deemed to be equipped to practise with safety and competence. It also indicates that, while some developments in midwifery become an essential and integral part of the role of every midwife (and are subsequently incorporated into pre-registration education), other developments may require particular midwives to acquire new skills because of the particular settings in which they are practising. The importance of local policies which are in accord with the Council's policies and standards and the guidelines issued by the National Boards for Nursing, Midwifery and Health Visiting is self-evident. The importance of the midwife practising outside the area of her employing authority or outside the National Health Service discussing the full scope of her practice with her supervisor of midwives is emphasised in the Midwife's Code of Practice.

(16) It can be seen from this position that it is accepted by the Council that some developments in midwifery care can become an integral part of the role of all midwives and other developments may become part of the role of some midwives. The Council believes that the Midwife's Code of Practice, cited above, and the Code of Professional Conduct, together provide key principles to underpin the scope of midwifery practice. These are now supplemented by those stated in paragraphs 8 to 10 inclusive of this paper.

The Scope of Health Visiting Practice

(17) The position of health visiting differs from that of nursing and midwifery, as there are frequent occasions when the full contribution of health visitors may not find expression where it is most needed. There is, for example, often a concentration on the role of the health visitor in relation to those in the under-five age group at the expense of other groups in the community who need, and would benefit from, the special preparation and skill of health visitors. These circumstances have the effect of constraining practice and limiting the degree to which individuals and communities are able to benefit from the knowledge and skill of health visitors. There is merit in allowing health visitors, where they judge it to be appropriate, to use the full range of their skills in response to needs identified in the pursuit of their health visiting practice. To single out any aspect of practice would be unwise but, where health and nursing need is identified, the health visitor is well placed to determine

what intervention may be necessary and able to draw on both her nursing and health visiting education.

(18)   The community setting of health visiting practice, the relationship between numerous agencies and services and the health visitor's professional relationship with clients and their families are factors which must be taken into consideration. The health visitor, in all aspects of her practice, is subject to the Council's Code of Professional Conduct and should also satisfy the requirements of paragraphs 8 to 10 inclusive of this paper.

Practice and the 'Identified' Nurse, Midwife and Health Visitor

(19)   The Council recognises that, in a growing number of settings, patients and clients will be in the care of an 'identified' practitioner. The practitioner may be identified as the 'named' practitioner or as the primary, associate or sole practitioner providing nursing, midwifery or health visiting care. In such roles, individuals assume key responsibility for coordinating and supervising the delivery of care, drawing on the general and special resources of colleagues where appropriate. Professional practice naturally involves recognising and accepting accountability for these matters. The Council expects that practitioners will recognise the need to provide all necessary support for colleagues and ensure that practice is underpinned by the required knowledge and skill. The Council equally expects that practitioners identified in one of these ways will be fully prepared for, and supported, in this key role.

Practice in the Personal Social Services and Residential Care Sector

(20)   The Council recognises that the community nursing services have a duty to provide a nursing service to those in need of nursing care in the personal social services and residential care sector. Registered nurses who are employed in this sector, whether in homes or in the provision of other services, remain accountable to the Council and subject to the Council's Code of Professional Conduct, even if their posts do not require nursing qualifications. In this regard, as explained in paragraph 5 of this paper, the position of such nurses is the same as that of nurses engaged in direct professional nursing practice.

(21)   The Council requires that registered nurses employed in such circumstances will use their judgement and discretion to identify the nursing needs of residents and others for whom they may have responsibility, and will comply with any requirements of the Council. The Council expects that employers will recognise the advantages to the personal social services and residential care sector which result from the employment of registered nurses.

Support for Professional Practice

(22)   Nurses, midwives and health visitors require support in their work. In institutional and community settings, a range of support staff form part of the team. The development of the health care assistant role is linked with a form of vocational training. The Council does not have a direct role in this training, but recognises that this development has an impact upon aspects of care and on the practice and standards of nursing, midwifery and health visiting, for which the Council is responsible.

(23)   The Council's position in relation to support roles is as follows:
   23.1   health care assistants to registered nurses, midwives and health visitors must work under the direction and supervision of those registered practitioners;
   23.2   registered nurses, midwives and health visitors must remain accountable for

assessment, planning and standards of care and for determining the activity of their support staff;

23.3   health care assistants must not be allowed to work beyond their level of competence;

23.4   continuity of care and appropriate skill/staff mix is important, so health care assistants should be integral members of the caring team;

23.5   standards of care must be safeguarded and the need for patients and clients across the spectrum of health care, to receive skilled professional nursing, midwifery and health visiting assessment and care must be recognised as of primary importance;

23.6   health care assistants with the desire and ability to progress to professional education should be encouraged to obtain vocational qualifications, some of which may be approved by the Council as acceptable entry criteria into programmes of professional education and

23.7   registered nurses, midwives and health visitors should be involved in these developments so that the support role can be designed to ensure that professional skills are used most appropriately for the benefit of patients and clients.

Conclusion

(24)   The principles set out in paragraph 8 to 10 inclusive of this paper should form the basis for any decisions relating to adjustments to the scope of practice. These principles should replace the system of certification for specific tasks. They provide a realistic, effective and rational approach to adjustments to professional practice.

(25)   This change has consequences for managers of clinical practice and professional leaders of nursing, midwifery and health visiting, who must ensure that local policies and procedures are based upon the principles set out in this paper and in the Council's Code of Professional Conduct. Any local arrangements must ensure that registered nurses, midwives and health visitors are assisted to undertake, and are enabled to fulfil, any suitable adjustments to their scope of practice.

(26)   This statement sets out the Council's position relating to the scope of professional practice of the professions it regulates, to the 'identified' practitioner, to practice in the residential care sector and to support staff. The Council hopes that this statement, and the principles which it sets out, will provide a clear framework for the logical and desirable development of practice and for the management of practice and care teams. The framework provides for greater flexibility in practice and for enhancing the contribution to care of nurses, midwives and health visitors. Above all, the framework and the principles reflect the personal responsibility and accountability of individual practitioners, entrusted by the Council to protect and improve standards of care.

(27)   Enquiries in respect of this Council paper should be directed to the:

Registrar and Chief Executive
United Kingdom Central Council
for Nursing, Midwifery and Health Visiting
23 Portland Place
London
W1N 3AF

Appendix II
Report of the Advisory Group on Nurse Prescribing
Department of Health, December 1989

Core Recommendations

Summary
This report recommends that certain groups of nurses working in the community should be authorised to prescribe from a limited list of products and to supply medicines, to vary their timing and dosage, within agreed protocols. It puts forward proposals for the introduction of nurse prescribing and suggests a timetable for the necessary education and training of nurses and for the legislative changes that will be required.

The recommendations are addressed to the Department of Health, to the professions, to the United Kingdom Central Council for Nursing, Midwifery and Health Visiting (UKCC), and to health authorities.

I. **The** *core recommendations* are:

Recommendation 1 (Chapter 1, paragraph 1.22)
Suitably qualified nurses working in the community (as defined below) should be able, in clearly defined circumstances, to prescribe from a limited list of items and to adjust the timing and dosage of medicines within a set protocol.

Recommendation 2 (Chapter 2, paragraph 2.3)
Certain specified groups of nurses should be able to:
- *prescribe* from a Nurses' Formulary (initial prescribing);
- *supply* within a group protocol agreed for a particular clinical service. The protocol should include arrangements for initial assessment and review;
- *adjust* the timing and dosage of medicines within a patient-specific protocol.

Recommendation 3 (Chapter 3)
Nurses with a district nurse or health visitor qualification (including those employed as paediatric community nurses, practice nurses or private nurses – paragraph 3.5), having had the necessary additional training:
  (i)   should be empowered to *prescribe* items necessary for the care of patients with those conditions for which the nurse takes independent clinical responsibility (paragraph 3.4);
  (ii) should be able to *supply* certain categories of patients with items within a group protocol and adjust the timing and dosage of medicines within a patient-specific protocol (paragraphs 3.10–3.12).

Recommendation 4 (Chapter 3, paragraph 3.10)
Supply within a group protocol. In addition to nurses with a district nurse or health visitor qualification, certain groups of nurses who have successfully completed the appropriate specialist education, training and assessment should be able to *supply* certain categories of patients with items within a group protocol. At present, we recommend that stoma care nurses, continence advisers, school nurses and paediatric clinical nurse specialists should be given this authority.

Recommendation 5 (Chapter 3, paragraph 3.12)
Adjusting timing and dosage of medicines. In addition to nurses with a district nurse or health visitor qualification, certain community nursing staff who have successfully completed appropriate specialist education, training and assessment should be able within a *patient-specific* protocol to adjust the timing and dosage of medicines which are prescribed by medical practitioners. At present we propose that community psychiatric nurses, community mental handicap nurses, specialist nurses for terminally ill patients and diabetic liaison nurses should be given this authority.

Recommendation 30 (Chapter 10, paragraphs 10.2–10.4)
An appropriate timetable for the introduction of nurse prescribing should be set nationally in consultation with potential nurse prescribers and taking account of education and training requirements. The legislative and education/training timetables should be co-ordinated. The aim should be to introduce nurse prescribing on 1 April 1992.

II The following recommendations are addressed to the *Department of Health:*

Recommendation 9 (Chapter 4, paragraph 4.10)
A Nurses' Formulary should be drawn up by the Department of Health, in consultation with the appropriate professions, to include the groups of medicines, dressings and appliances, and diagnostic agents set out in Appendix E.

Recommendation 29 (Chapter 8, paragraph 8.6)
The necessary legislative changes should be made as soon as possible in order to enable nurses with district nurse and health visitor qualifications to prescribe all the items in the Nurses' Formulary.

Recommendation 10 (Chapter 4, paragraph 4.11)
The Nurses' Formulary should be reviewed regularly, taking account of appropriate professional advice.

Recommendation 25 (Chapter 7, paragraph 7.15)
Prescription pads printed on distinctive paper should be issued to authorised nurse prescribers working in the NHS and include the name, qualifications, professional address and telephone number of the prescriber.

Recommendation 26 (Chapter 7, paragraph 7.16)
Prescriptions issued by nurses working outside the NHS should carry the name, qualifications, professional address and telephone number of the prescriber.

Recommendation 31 (Chapter 10, paragraph 10.8)
An evaluation programme should be established before the implementation of nurse prescribing so that some relevant baseline information can be gathered.

Recommendation 32 (Chapter 10, paragraph 10.8)
The evaluation study should include an assessment of the views of patients, relatives, nurses and other members of primary health care teams, as well as a full economic appraisal. Where possible, health outcomes should be measured.

Recommendation 6 (Chapter 3, paragraph 3.9)
Further consideration should be given, in the light of experience, to extending initial prescribing authority to some other groups of specialist nurses.

Recommendation 7 (Chapter 3, paragraph 3.16)
The groups of specialist nurses identified in recommendations 4 and 5 as authorised to supply items, or adjust the timing and dosage of medicines, should be reviewed from time to time to take account of changes in clinical practice, and the role of family planning nurses should be considered in this context.

III   The following recommendations are addressed to the *professions*:

Recommendation 14 (Chapter 6, paragraphs 6.1 and 6.5)
Good communications between health professionals and patients, and between different professionals, are essential for high quality health care. All health professionals empowered to prescribe for a patient should have access to the relevant patient records.

Recommendation 19 (Chapter 6, paragraphs 6.12 and 6.13)
Patients' personal record cards showing the timing and dosage of all medication, and other relevant information, should be completed by each professional who prescribes for the patients and updated to show any changes. These should be available to doctors and nurses treating the patient and to pharmacists issuing medicines. Patient-held records of medication should be used wherever possible.

Recommendation 16 (Chapter 6, paragraph 6.10)
'Patient-specific protocols' should be drawn up by all the practitioners responsible for the care of the patient. These protocols must be written, with copies in the patient's records and available to all authorised prescribers for the patient and to pharmacists, as necessary.

Recommendation 17 (Chapter 6, paragraph 6.11)
In the event of a disagreement between professionals over the treatment of a patient, the general practitioner (GP) responsible for the care of the patient will, as at present, take the final decision.

Recommendation 18 (Chapter 6, paragraph 6.11)
The pharmacist must retain the right not to dispense a prescription on professional grounds.

Recommendation 8 (Chapter 3, paragraph 3.17)
A nurse who accepts a post for which the ability to prescribe, supply or adjust the timing and dosage of medicines is a requirement set out in the job description will be expected to accept this responsibility.

Recommendation 22 (Chapter 7, paragraph 7.6)
It should be the responsibility of each nurse to ensure that her qualifications are registered or recorded with the UKCC. The employing authority, and others involved in agreeing protocols, must make sure that she has done so.

IV   The following recommendations are addressed to the *UKCC and National Boards for Nursing, Midwifery and Health Visiting*:

Recommendation 11 (Chapter 5, paragraph 5.5)
The UKCC should be invited to devise a policy aimed at ensuring that all nurses currently holding district nurse and health visitor qualifications receive such additional education, training and assessment as will enable them to demonstrate to a National Board for Nursing, Midwifery and Health Visiting adequate knowledge of pharmacology and therapeutics relevant to the products which they may subsequently be authorised to prescribe.

Recommendation 12 (Chapter 5, paragraphs 5.6 and 5.9)
In future, all post-registration courses in health visiting and district nursing should include tuition and assessment to a level to be determined by the National Boards in pharmacology, therapeutics and practical prescribing. The present courses for continence advisers and specialist diabetic liaison nurses should be extended to include these subjects.

Recommendation 13 (Chapter 5, paragraph 5.10)
The UKCC and National Boards should be responsible for all aspects of policy in relation to nurse education and training, and for the provision of formal courses. No events wholly arranged or resourced by commercial companies should be recognised for formal training purposes.

Recommendation 20 (Chapter 7, paragraphs 7.3 and 7.4)
The UKCC should be asked to continue to identify nurses with district nurse and health visitor qualifications on its register, and to indicate which of those nurses have completed the necessary additional education and training to enable them to prescribe.

Recommendation 21 (Chapter 7, paragraph 7.6)
The UKCC should make the information on its register of nurse prescribers available to *bona fide* enquirers.

V The following recommendations are addressed to *health authorities and Family Practitioner Committees (FPCs)*:

Recommendation 28 (Chapter 7, paragraph 7.11)
Each authorised nurse prescriber working in the NHS should have an honorary contract with the appropriate FPC.

Recommendation 15 (Chapter 6, paragraph 6.10)
In every health authority, a group protocol agreed for a particular clinical service should be drawn up by those responsible for service delivery, using a working group which includes representatives of the doctors, nurses and pharmacists involved. The protocols must be written, regularly reviewed and issued to all relevant health professionals.

Recommendation 23 (Chapter 7, paragraph 7.6)
The employing authority should maintain records of authorised nurse prescribers in its employment.

Recommendation 24 (Chapter 7, paragraph 7.14)
Nurse precribers should be provided with regular reports on their prescribing patterns.

Recommendation 27 (Chapter 7, paragraph 7.18)
Health authorities should set up practicable systems in their own areas for the supply of single doses of some products, where appropriate, and to provide nurses with their necessary basic supplies.

Post-Registration Education and Practice Project (PREPP) Report (UKCC) 1990

Resume of Recommendations

(1) There should be a period of support for all newly registered practitioners to consolidate the competencies or learning outcomes achieved at registration.

(2) A preceptor should provide the support for each newly registered practitioner.

(3) All nurses, midwives and health visitors must demonstrate that they have maintained and developed their professional knowledge and competence.

(4) All practitioners must record their professional development in a personal professional profile.

(5) During the 3 years leading to periodic registration, all practitioners must complete a period of study or provide evidence of appropriate professional learning. A minimum of 5 days of study leave every 3 years must be undertaken by every registered practitioner.

(6) When registered practitioners wish to return to practice after a break of 5 years or more, they will have to complete a return to practice programme.

(7) The standard, kind and content of preparation for specialist enhanced practice will be specified by the Council. Definition of enhanced specialist and advanced practitioners are stated.

(8) To be eligible to practise, individuals must every 3 years: submit a notification of practice; *either* provide verification that they have completed their personal professional profile satisfactorily; *or* show evidence that they have completed a return to practice programme; and pay their periodic fee.

(9) Practitioners after a break of less than 5 years returning to practice using a specific registered qualification shall submit a notification of practice and, within the following calendar year, provide verification that they have completed their personal professional profile satisfactorily.

Appendix IV
Training for Accident and Emergency Nursing

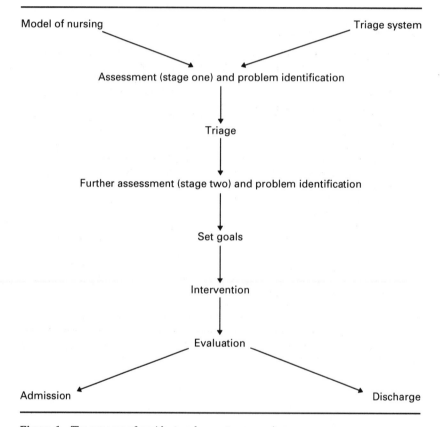

Model of nursing

Triage system

Assessment (stage one) and problem identification

Triage

Further assessment (stage two) and problem identification

Set goals

Intervention

Evaluation

Admission

Discharge

Figure 1   The process of accident and emergency nursing care.

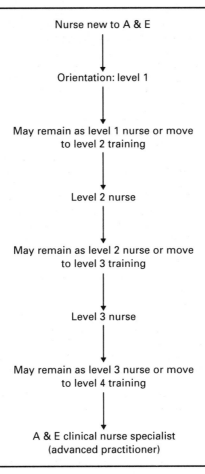

Figure 2 Accident and emergency nursing development programme (from novice to clinical specialist).

This level one package prepares the new nurse to A & E to practise competently as an associate nurse within the A & E department.

(1) The model of nursing.
(2) Interpersonal skills 1, including:
Bereavement suport and the issues surrounding sudden death and sudden infant death syndrome.
Handling the violent and potentially violent patient 1, for example ENB Course 955 Handling the violent and potentially violent patient.
(3) Care of the patient with major injuries.
(4) Care of the patient with chest pain 1 and breathing difficulties 1, including recording and interpretation of the ECG. Basic cardio-pulmonary resuscitation and administration of oxygen.
(5) Care of the patient with a limb injury, including the application of bandages, strapping and plaster of Paris.
(6) Care of the patient with a wound 1, including tetanus toxoid administration, various wound dressings and the application of glue.
(7) Care of the patient who has taken a drugs overdose including the technique of stomach lavage.
(8) Care of the mentally disturbed patient 1: the Mental Health Act and dealing with patients who have behavioural problems and/or are under the influence of alcohol and/or drugs.
(9) Correct assessment and intervention of patients arriving in the department, including blood sugar estimation, routine observations, airway management, administration of IV drugs, etc.
(10) Law and ethics 1, including the collection of forensic evidence.
(11) Health and safety issues, including infection control and the contaminated patient.
(12) Care of the patient in pain, including the role and use of Entonox.
(13) Care of the child 1, including recognition of child abuse and intervention.
(14) Care of the frail elderly.
(15) The nurse's role in the pre-hospital environment, including practical experience with an ambulance crew.
(16) The nurse's role during a major disaster, including chemical and radiation incidents.
(17) The role of social services, social workers, police and other support professions.
(18) Observation of triage.

Figure 3 Level one training.

This level prepares the nurse to practise competently as a primary nurse within the A & E department

(1) Triage training, including further development of the nurse's interpersonal skills.
(2) Becoming the named nurse, role development.
(3) The nurse as the supervisor of a clinical area.
(4) Care of the patient with a wound 2, including the technique of skin suturing and the use of local anaesthesia.
(5) Care of the patient with major injuries 2, including advanced life-support skills. The nurse should attend an advanced trauma course.
(6) Care of the patient with chest pain 2, including defibrillation.
(7) Development of the role nurses play in health promotion and environmental safety guidance.
(8) Use of research 1 and how to support research in the department.
(9) How to mentor junior nurses, including attendance at ENB course 998 Teaching and Assessing.
(10) Emergency child birth and care of the newborn.
(11) Care of the violent patient 2.
(12) Care of the mentally disturbed patient 2, including specific training in liaison with the psychiatric unit.
(13) Care of the child 2, including specific training in liaison with the paediatric unit.
(14) Care of the frail elderly 2, including specific training in liaison with the care of the elderly unit and social services.
(15) Law and ethics 2.

Figure 4 Level 2 training.

This level is designed to prepare the nurse to work as an emergency nurse practitioner and shift coordinator.

(1) Attend an in-house course for nurse practitioners or a course run by another hospital or institution.
(2) Develop further research skills.
(3) Develop counselling skills/crisis intervention skills.
(4) Attend management study days and courses.
(5) Training to be provided for the role of department shift coordinator.
(6) Evaluate new equipment and prepare information for staff.
(7) Law and ethics 3.

Figure 5 Level 3 training.

This level provides the nurse with the appropriate additional knowledge to act as a clinical nurse specialist within the A & E speciality.

The nurse on completion of this level should be able to:

(1) Explain scientific foundations underlying the management of patients with traumatic, medical and surgical conditions.
(2) Discuss new developments in A & E care.
(3) Assess the physical, psychological and social needs of patients and their relatives.
(4) Discuss the psychological effects of A & E work upon the staff working in the speciality and intervene as necessary.
(5) Discuss in depth the ethical and legal aspects of A & E work.
(6) Demonstrate his/her ability to carry out research within the department.
(7) Demonstrate an in-depth knowledge of quality, standards and audit.
(8) Manage the department including staff appraisal, interviewing, etc.

Figure 6   Level 4 training.

Appendix V

The Extending Role of the Nurse

(Department of Health and Social Security), September 1989

PL/CMO(89)7 and PL/CNO(89)10

Note: This document was withdrawn by the Health Departments in July 1992 and is superseded by the UKCC's *The Scope of Professional Practice* (Appendix I in this volume). We include it here for historical interest. Earlier documents on role extension which have also been withdrawn are: in June 1977 Department of Health (England) letter CMO(77)10/CNO(77)9 accompanied by health circular HC77(22) and in Wales CMO(77)10/CNO(77)15 and health circular WHC(77)25; in 1983 the Northern Ireland Department of Health and Social Services circular HSS(TH)1/83.

The extending role of the nurse

Report of a Working Party set up jointly by the Standing Medical Advisory Committee and the Standing Nursing and Midwifery Advisory Committee

Background

(3) Guidance on the extending role of the clinical nurse was issued in Health Circular (77)22. This guidance recognised that in both primary and specialist health care, nurses had become increasingly involved in tasks, procedures and decision making, which had previously been a medical responsibility. It saw this trend as being the result of a number of factors, including the increasing complexity of treatment and the growth in the specialist expertise of the nurse. The circular welcomed this trend, and gave guidance on the procedures to be followed in the delegation of activities by doctors to nurses and on the prerequisite qualifications of the individual nurse.

(4) The circular was concerned only with the relationship between the medical and nursing profession, and only with nurses employed by health authorities. No mention was made of the delegation of tasks to nurses by members of other health professions, of delegation within the nursing profession, of the special position of midwives, or of nurses outside health authority employ.

(5) The guidance was generally welcomed at the time as providing a sensible framework within which the nurse's role might be extended. It facilitated the flexible and efficient provision of patient care, allowing doctors greater freedom in the allocation of their time and increasing the job satisfaction of nurses. Since then, however, a number of difficulties have arisen or become apparent:

    (i) The Circular assumed that policies for extending the nurse's role would be initiated by health authorities, but health authorities are remote from the clinical context where delegation occurs and this assumption constrains the scope for initiatives;

    (ii) There is inconsistency in the practice of delegation both between and within health authorities;

    (iii) There is inconsistency in the recognition of the training appropriate for nurses who are to perform delegated tasks; we are aware of instances of nurses being required to repeat training courses that they have already attended when employed elsewhere, and, which is more serious, of nurses receiving cursory training or training inadequate for their individual needs;

    (iv)   There is no consensus within the professions nationally as to which tasks fall appropriately within the nurse's extending roles.

(6)   We believe that extending the nurse's role remains crucial to the provision and development of patient care. In our view the principles established in HC(77)22 remain essentially sound, but they need to be re-interpreted and re-expressed in the light of developments in clinical practice and changes in health service organisation, if nurses are to continue to use their skills and resources in the most effective way. In particular, attention needs to be given to the Nurses, Midwives and Health Visitors Rules Approval Order 1983 (SI 1983/783) made under the Nurses, Midwives and Health Visitors Act 1979, which sets out the differences between the competencies required of first level nurses (eg RGN, RMN, RNMH, RSCN) and those required of second level nurses (i.e. enrolled nurses). Attention should also be given to the UKCC Code of Professional Conduct which sets out the professional accountability of each registered nurse, midwife and health visitor.

(7)   In the paragraphs that follow we examine the context in which the nurse's role is extending. Whereas HC(77)22 used the word 'tasks', we prefer to use the word 'activities', since the former implies a task-oriented approach to the provision of care which we would not necessarily wish to encourage; we support the concept of the nurse's concern being for the patient as a whole person. As required by our terms of reference, we confine our recommendations to the relationship between the medical and nursing professions, we do not refer to nurses outside health authority employ, and we make no reference to practising midwives who are subject to their own rules and Code of Practice. We recognise, however, that practice nurses, occupational health nurses, school health nurses employed by education authorities, and nurses employed in nursing homes registered with health authorities, also perform tasks delegated by doctors, and in our view the principles recommended in the guidance could provide a helpful framework for such delegation. As is explained in para 10 we have not addressed the matter of the nurse specialist. Our remit extends only to England and Wales.

(8)   The personal pronouns used in this report assume that doctors are male and nurses female. This is purely a matter of linguistic convenience; we recognise that many doctors are female and many nurses male, and we apologise if our language gives any offence.

The definition of activities

(9)   HC(77)22 appreciates that the boundary line between those activities that fall within the traditional role of the nurse and those that are undertaken by the nurse as an extension of that role is not fixed for all time; what is expected of nurses is constantly changing and developing. We think it is helpful to define the activities of nurses in terms of three categories:

    (i)   Those activities for which nurses are prepared in the course of their pre-registration training;

    (ii)   Those more specialised activities for which nurses are prepared by post-registration training. These include those activities undertaken in the community, by for example health visitors, district nurses and community psychiatric nurses.

    (iii)   Activities normally undertaken by doctors but which may be delegated in appropriate circumstances, and which may be performed by nurses with appropriate training and competence.

(10) Post-certificate courses organised by the English and Welsh National Boards prepare nurses for activities that fall within the second and third categories, but it is only the third category that represents the extending area of the nurse's role. In our view the role of nurse specialists, their relationships with doctors and other health professionals and the legal implications of their extending role require more careful scrutiny; we have not considered it in this report.

(11) We wish to emphasise that the nurse's primary obligation is to the performance of nursing activities that fall within her customary professional role, i.e. within the first two categories. While we welcome the extension of that role in appropriate circumstances, we would not wish it to happen at the expense of the performance of the nurse's customary activities.

(12) HC(77)22 requires that the tasks performed by nurses extending their role should be 'recognised by the professions', and we agree with this requirement. However, we do not consider it practicable for the professions to promulgate a national list of specific activities that are appropriate for delegation. Such a list could never be comprehensive and would require frequent updating and a national list would militate against the development of methods of working which are appropriate in some local circumstances but not in others. We are aware of activities carried out by specially trained nurses at specialist units with the approval of the health authority concerned and while we have no reason to doubt the appropriateness of such delegation in particular circumstances, it would not be appropriate to encourage from the centre such practice elsewhere in the absence of particular knowledge of working methods and staffing. We recommend instead that the activities that are appropriate for delegation by doctors to nurses in a particular care setting and speciality should be agreed by the medical and nursing professions locally.

Local policies

(13) HC(77)22 requires that the tasks performed by nurses extending their role be recognised by their employing authority, and we see it as essential that, because of the liability of her employing authority for a nurse's actions, the extension would happen only within the context of a policy that the employing authority has approved. In the course of such approval being given we would expect the general manager to take advice from the health authority's medical and nursing advisors, and to take legal advice where necessary. There are clear advantages in policies being coordinated throughout the health authority, and we would expect the general manager to take these into account. It is, however, equally important that particular policies should be agreed by the medical and nursing professions within the relevant units or departments.

(14) In our view the most likely method for establishing a policy will be as follows:

(i) The initiative will probably be taken in the ward or clinical department where the delegated activities are to be performed by the professional staff concerned;

(ii) The suggested policy will then be discussed locally and referred to the professional representative structures;

(iii) The suggested policy, when professionally agreed, will then be submitted to the District for health authority approval. Where nurses are to perform delegated activities beyond the geographical boundaries of their employing authority, the other health authorities concerned will need to be informed and their consent obtained;

(iv) Copies of the approved policy will then be made available to the unit general manager, to the professional representative bodies, within the District, and to all the doctors and nurses who will be involved in its implementation.

These procedures will ensure that policies for the delegation of activities are rooted in a practical understanding of the clinical tasks that need to be performed, are agreed between the professions at District level, are approved by the employing authority, and are promulgated and properly understood.

The nurse's training and competence

(15) HC(77)22 requires that the nurse has been 'specifically and adequately trained for the task', that 'the training has been recognised as satisfactory by her employing authority', and that the 'delegating doctor has been assured of the competence of the individual nurse concerned'. The importance of the individual nurse being both trained and competent goes without saying.

(16) The English and Welsh National Boards' approved courses provide training in nursing activities which fall within the nurse's extended role. We recommend that the successful completion of such a course in recent or current clinical practice be recognised as evidence of adequate training by all health authorities and by all doctors and nurses involved in the delegation of relevant activities. We appreciate, however, that these National Board courses do not cover all the activities that may be appropriate for delegation, and we recognise that it is sometimes necessary for training courses to be organised at district or unit level, or for individual training to be provided within the relevant clinical environment. We see it as the responsibility of the senior nurse/ward sister to assess the training requirements of each individual nurse, taking account of the nurse's previous experience and of the quality and content of any previous training, and then to ensure that the nurse receives training appropriate for the activities that are to be performed.

(17) HC(77)22 requires that the nurse be not only trained but also competent. While we see the recognition of training completed as being transferrable from one clinical situation to another, we recommend that each nurse's competence be assessed in each new clinical environment before she starts to perform particular delegated activities. This assessment would normally be made by the clinical nurse to whom she is accountable, but in certain circumstances might more appropriately be made by the relevant consultant or general practitioner. The form that the assessment would take would vary according to the nature of the activities and the nurse's training and previous experience, and on some occasions a brief period of supervision might be sufficient. We recommend that when a nurse has been assessed as competent in the performance of particular activities, this be recorded in her personal file and a written note of it made readily available on her ward or clinical department.

The nurse's consent

(18) HC(77)22 requires that a nurse who performs a task as an extension of her role 'agrees to undertake it'. This requirement remains essential, and nurses should not be put under pressure to agree against their will or better judgement and should be free to withdraw their agreement if they so choose, giving reasonable notice. If the performance of such activities is a requirement of any particular post, we recommend that a nurse be asked for her agreement before being appointed to the post, and that this agreement be recorded in her letter of appointment. It should be remembered that a nurse's primary commitment is to the performance of activities that fall within her customary role.

The enrolled nurse

(19) By the Nurses, Midwives and Health Visitors Rules Approval Order 1983 (SI 1983/667), made under the Nurses, Midwives and Health Visitors Act 1979, the Register is divided into 11 Parts. Parts 2, 3, 5 and 8 of the register comprise 'first level' nurses

and Parts 2, 4, 6 and 7 of the register comprise 'second level' nurses (Part 9, Nurses trained in the nursing of patients suffering from fever, Part 10, Midwives and Part 11, Health Visitors fall outside this distinction). The qualifications held by 'first level' nurses are Registered General Nurse (previously known as SRN – State Registered Nurse), Registered Mental Nurse, Registered Nurse Mental Handicap and Registered Sick Children's Nurse while 'second level' nurses are those qualified as Enrolled Nurses. The Nurse, Midwives and Health Visitors Rules Approval Order 1983 (SI 1983/873) sets out the training leading to admission to the various parts. Rule 18 makes clear that the competencies required from those who successfully complete courses leading to admission to those parts of the register related to first level nurses and those parts related to second level nurses are different; in particular, that preparation for second level nursing prepares the student '. . . to undertake nursing care under the direction of a person registered in Part 1, 3, 5 or 8 of the Register'.

(20) There may be no objection to second level nurses (enrolled nurses) performing activities which extend their role, provided that the nurses have been given the necessary training and achieved the necessary level of competence under the direction of an appropriate first level nurse. However, it would not be in accordance with the statutory instrument to give *unqualified* approval to direct delegation from doctors to second level nurses. It is essential that when doctors and nurse managers are considering the delegation of activities to second level, enrolled nurses and when health authorities are considering policies that involve delegation, proper recognition is given to the nature of the training that second level nurses have received and consequently their particular training needs.

Liability

(21) In any action for damages, a nurse may be held legally liable if it can be shown either that she has failed to exercise skills properly expected of her or that she has undertaken activities she was not competent to perform. A doctor may be held legally liable if it can be shown that he has delegated to a nurse activities which were either outside the scope of the duties she was normally expected to perform, or in which she was not adequately trained or competent. We are advised that recommendations we have made provide an adequate basis for the performance by nurses of activities delegated to them by doctors. In approving policies for the extension of the nurse's role, the health authority would accept liability for the nurse's actions; we understand that Departmental and Regional lawyers unanimously agree that the usual arrangements by which health authorities indemnify employees would cover all extended activities undertaken in the course of employment.

Index